What other read

"Eating After Eden............ .... teaching into applicable day-to-day guidelines for the modern audience that wishes to seek enhanced health in a fallen world.

"Many of the premature deaths that befall the western world could be averted if everyone who wants to bestow the ultimate gift would share this book with friends and family. "

Chris D. Meletis, ND
Physician
Oregon

* * * * * * *

"Through the years, my almost-daily contact with Dr. Zook has rewarded me with observation of her passion for true health, nutritional sense for suffering bodies, and spiritual wisdom for lost souls.

"Our modern culture has departed from the original, fundamental principles of diet for achieving health. *Eatin' After Eden* provides the truth about what foods should be present in our 21st Century diet for physical well-being to the end of our appointed days."

Jerry Linnenkohl, BS
Nutritionist
Washington

* * * * * * *

"I am going through *Eatin after Eden'* very slowly. I did not expect that I would be reading it like I am. I normally cruise through books, even complex books, pretty quickly. However, I...am reading sentence by sentence, letting it all soak in...

"[As a former school teacher] if it were up to me this would be required reading in the schools at a very, very early age. It's so important *right now*. I can't say enough positive things about what I have read so far.

"You make a very compelling argument against vegetarian and veganism. I can't imagine anyone reading those chapters and thinking that either of those two alternatives are what our Creator intended for us.

"You also raise thought-provoking questions, such as the one about the association of soy, thyroid and cancer. In fact, **one of the things I really enjoy about your book is that you ask questions of the reader all along, causing them to stop and *think*...** you have taught me to think critically in regard to health.

"The book answers the question of how modern man has gotten into the terrible shape we are in - both physically and spiritually.

"Another illumination is that there is another 'way' of looking at our many problems than those recommendations given to us by the main stream.

These are a few of the many, many things I have learned from you. "I can't even begin to say how important your work is. We all need this now, ASAP! Sitting in a public place today I got a chance to see society. We need help! Folks just don't look well. I wanted to say, "I have this book you MUST read!"... Thanks for all you are doing. Great, great work."

Bob VanDeusen, BA
Real Estate Broker
Oregon

* * * * * * *

"In *Eatin' After Eden*, Dr. Zook scripturally, scientifically, and logically brings us back to what our Creator intended: foods that are critical to a powerful and sustaining diet. If only such a book had been available during my seven years as a struggling vegan (convinced as I was that veganism was "God's Ideal Diet"). It would have been more valuable to me than any amount of gold."

Greg Westbrook, MS
Electrical Engineer
Arizona

"Congratulations on *one of the most important books ever written for this end-time!* You have given us essential truths from God's Word and nutrition science that many physicians don't have, even good Christian "health doctors." Thanks for your time, experience, and expertise…The Church needs this *now!*"

John P. Rothacker, D.D.S.
Dentist & Author
Ohio

EATIN' AFTER EDEN

Sylvia W. Zook, MS, PhD

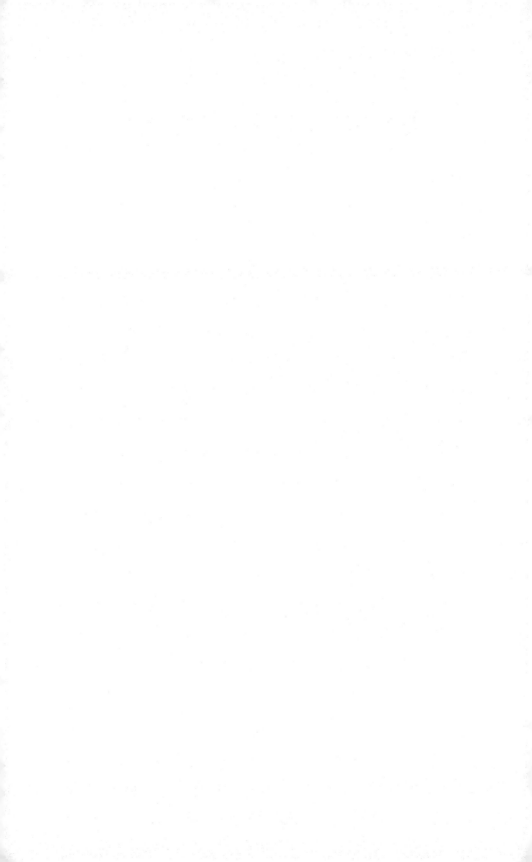

The Plumb Line

A plumb line or plummet is a weight with a pointed tip, suspended from a string, and used as a reference line that is perpendicular to the ground. Carpenters and bricklayers have used this same instrument since the time of the ancients, to ensure their constructions are both square and upright to the ground.

In the Bible, Zerubabel laid out the foundation of the Temple, using a plummet. He and Amos (a farmer) were also used as God's spiritual "plumb lines" to help Jehovah's people get back in line with His Word.

America has veered far from the Creator's post-Edenic dietary "blueprint" with profoundly tragic consequences of myriad kinds. The well-referenced,[1] scientifically based "plumb line" you hold in your hand, reveals His nutrition plan as found in His Word from Genesis to Revelation. May He grant you the capacity to discern His loving heart as manifested by that and post-Eden nutritional gifts - indispensable gifts to His children seeking to obey Him in all things, for their good and His glory.

---

[1] Though it requires extensive labor, we have chosen to place the documentation and commentary at the bottom of the page for the reader's convenience, rather than as endnotes at the back of the book.

EATIN' AFTER EDEN

Sylvia W. Zook, MS, PhD

Plumb Line Publisher
Salem, Oregon

Disclaimer: This book is intended solely for educational purposes, and nothing in this book is intended as medical counseling. The reader fully understands that no statement in this book is meant to discourage anyone from following one's physician's advice. No one should discontinue prescription medications without the advice of same. This book neither suggests nor implies that services of medical practitioners be replaced. No statement, food, or product mentioned in this book is intended to diagnose, prescribe, treat, prevent, or cure disease. The mention of any resource in this book does not imply or constitute an endorsement or guarantee of its quality by the author. Further, the author specifically disclaims any and all liability for judgments, claims, costs, damages, or injuries from any products or resources mentioned by the author or offered by any of the sources as mentioned in this book. No recipe or food mentioned in this book is intended for use by those who may have an allergy, sensitivity, or intolerance to such foods. The reader understands that diet and lifestyle changes should be undertaken in consultation with one's physician.

Scripture references and quotations in this book are from the King James Bible unless otherwise noted.

Copyright © 2008, 2012 by Sylvia W. Zook, MS, PhD. All rights reserved. No part of this publication may be stored in a retrieval system, transmitted by any means, or reproduced in any way, including photocopying, except with the prior written permission of the author.

Revised edition 2012 and second printing.

Plumb Line Publisher, PO Box 3743, Salem, OR 97302
Printed in the United States of America

ISBN-13: 978-1468123043
ISBN-10: 1468123041
LCCN: 2008932739

This book is lovingly dedicated to Mother,
who first introduced me to nutrition science.
Thirty years later I returned it an enhanced gift
she says enabled her to live another 15 productive years.
Now well into her nineties, Mother has
has lived far longer than any other in her family.

Acknowledgements

After the divine commision to write this book, Father God sovreignly selected a support team. All through the work, I have been introduced to new friends and come to know old ones better, as we all have labored together in this part of His "vineyard" for this time.

First, Jehovah Jireh, our Provider, blessed this venture with three editors from diverse backgrounds for different tasks. All are highly skilled and experienced in their callings. Each immediately saw the urgent need for this book. They all have provided valuable, on-going, chapter-by-chapter commentary, undergirded by prayer. I was unaware at the time some of them came on board, that they too were published authors. However, Father knew and hand-picked them each.

Additionally, He knew all three were strong encouragers that would be needed in the incredibly grueling struggle ahead. I have not met one of them, and none has met the other editors. They are scattered over three states; yet amazingly, we have worked together as a team only the Spirit of God could have assembled.

First was Chris Meletis, ND, physician, colleague, and dear friend who reviewed the manuscript for medical accuracy and commentary in spite of his busy practice. Dr. Meletis has written 14 books and 200 white papers. He is much in demand as a nationally known lecturer.

Second, engineer Greg Westbrook, labored many hours with much patience, providing important editing. Greg's own book, *When Hallelujah Becomes"What Happened?"* tells of his family's frightening experience with veganism. His testimony is included herein.

Third, Joanne Krupp's reviewing the book for readability was a special blessing because she, unlike the others of the editorial team, had no nutrition educational background. Yet the Krupps were publishers for many years and have authored a number of books. They have been motivators with this and others of my works. A former school teacher, Joanne has provided good and practical pointers.

I could not have sat down and put together such a team as these four, who took time away from their busy lives and ministries to answer the call for this one. The Father who chose them will reward them eternally, of that I am certain.

Matt Stucker, a talented young writer, allowed me to "bounce" book and chapter names off him, with good suggestions. Bless you, Matt.

Val and Dick James have provided international soy information in heroic measure via their excellent website, SoyOnLineService. co.nz/ They have paid dearly for their courageous stand. The Jameses reviewed the soy chapter, *Why Not Soy Protein?*

Kaayla Daniel, PhD, also generously reviewed the soy chapter. Dr. Daniels has written the riveting work, *The Whole Soy Story* and serves on the Board of Directors for the Weston A. Price Foundation.

Sally Fallon Morell, President of the Weston A. Price Foundation, has always gotten back to me promptly with answers to questions regarding certain information at the magnificent website for the foundation. It provides abundant knowledge regarding traditional nutrition.

My family's patience and support have been crucial. Husband Ron took care of computer hardware, ran errands and handled many practical matters, freeing me to concentrate on research and countless studies, organizing materials, and writing. After a computer crash, son-in-law Doug (genius that he is) spent oodles of hours restoring countless research and manuscript files. Daughter Lori has always been there for encouragement, software issues, prayer support, graphic arts, and so very much more on a daily basis. Without her invaluable support, the book probably would still be just a vision.

From Genesis 3 when the serpent deceived Eve into believing that disobedience would make her wise, through the nutritional lie of the end time in 1 Timothy 4:3, God's plan for eating has been under attack by the adversary. Besides Scripture and real science supporting the truth of this book, concerted prayer has been a mainstay. I could not begin to name all who have been faithful with prayer support for this work the last couple of years. Again, God knows. Where He guided He has provided.

It is said that all researchers stand upon the shoulders of their predecessors. I am no different. I have labored to give credit to all those to whom we are indebted, hoping I have overlooked no one.

To all these I gratefully acknowledge the very important parts they have had in the creation of this educational tool. Already it has contributed to prevention of those conditions associated with inadequate nutrition, while supporting the body's continual healing of itself. This results in maintaining higher levels of wellness as designed by the Creator for His higher calling on the lives of each of us.

Contents

Introduction 16
How To Use This Book For Maximum Benefit 18
Chapter 1: The Fall – Before & After 21
Chapter 2: Eatin' After Eden - God's Awesome Gifts 29
Chapter 3: Quality Protein – The Best of the Story 39
Chapter 4: America's Rejection of God's Nutrition Plan 61
Chapter 5: It's In The Beef 105
Chapter 6: Protein Quality: God's Amazing "Gold Standard" 119
Chapter 7: Why Not Soy Protein? 135
Chapter 8: Vegetarianism – Is It Scientifically Sound? 155
Chapter 9: Veganism – Many "Spins," Same Sin 187
Chapter 10: Meat, Fish & Fowl - Should We Eat Them All? 237
Chapter 11: End Time Provision - Is It For Real? 249
Appendix A: Nutrients Required For Calcium Absorption 255
Appendix B: Pottenger's Cats 257
Appendix C: Bob & John's Garden–More Than It Appears 259
Recipes: Quickly Create Most Delicious, Healthiest Ones 261
Table of Acronyms 269
About the Author 271
Resources 273

Introduction

Over the years friends who are health care practitioners have expressed frustration and sadness in treating patients with certain conditions. These compassionate doctors lament the limitations for improvement when patient response to the standard of care is limited. In these cases, the aim becomes increased quality of life as patients must "learn to live with it."

In nutritional counseling and education those clients for me are long term vegans. Many of these describe themselves as "extremely health conscious," tell of their having cured themselves of serious health issues in years past, only to find that eventually they are unable to maintain an acceptable level of wellness, and their health is deteriorating. When presented with requirements for optimum nutrition, they balk. There is a check, a hindrance in their going forward. Usually their authoritative beliefs and philosophy will not allow change until they are desperate. I try to educate these nutritionally if they are open to it, and hope for the best. Yet I cannot heal anyone. The body requires certain nutrients in adequate amounts in order to carry on its work successfully. There is no sidestepping that.

With the dawning of the new millennium I became increasingly aware of the fast-growing numbers of another group of vegans within the Church. The enemy has placed another "spin" on this deficient diet based upon a huge limitation of Scripture. It troubles me because of my professional experience and knowledge of the ultimate consequences, no matter what one's religion. Out of deep concern this book was born.

First and foremost it identifies and explains scientifically and scripturally the critical nutritional value of the Creator's chief macronutrient of His gift and plan for eating after the Fall.

Secondly, the multiple deficiencies and profound consequences for the individual and nation in rejecting the divine plan are clearly defined. That rejection is usually manifested in following what was once called the Prudent Diet, as well as deceptive vegan diets to which even Christians are turning in alarming numbers today. If this book is a bit strong for some readers, please know that we have witnessed first hand what can happen when man's wisdom rejects God's. Not following the whole Word can be risky for us.

The American Church believes it may eat or *not* eat *any*thing it chooses. This includes "man-ufactured" non-foods, and other diets instead of the Creator's whole foods He designed for those He also created. His nutrition plan since the Fall is not debatable.[1] He does not leave us guessing, or to our own devices and wisdom.

In refusing to embrace the entire Scripture and interpreting it based upon man's changing philosophies, confusion is created. Thus saints put themselves at risk with potentially profound ramifications for themselves and succeeding generations. Such examples will be found in various chapters.

Dear reader, the point is that eating is major! All of our dietary liberty is within provided guidelines and principles. Should we arbitrarily decide how to eat anymore than we may worship, marry, make love, speak, work, and a host of other practices, based upon subjective preferences contrary to Scripture? Our loving Father has made it simple to please Him dietarily, and to enjoy a relatively high level of wellness as a result.

We are not saying that a carnal diet will send one to hell, however, the Bible says that those who live by the flesh will die by the flesh. In other words, there are consequences. We are to glorify God in all we do.

The thrust of this book is strongly scientific as well. Here you will learn of countless top researchers' studies, many of which only point to the import of that which God's Word has declared and instructed for thousands of years.

---

[1] For various reasons, there may individuals and special exceptions that prevent one from eating certain foods. We are dealing with general truth and principles here.

How To Use This Book For Maximum Benefit

Are you like me in that you like to open a book to the table of contents, then skip to certain chapters, quickly digesting a few rich morsels before settling in at the beginning? There's nothing wrong with that as long as you don't quickly page through "to get the gist of it," then put the book down, presuming to know and understand the writer's position on the subject. If you do that, you will have incomplete information. This book deals with complex matters of life and death. In addition to the "milk," much of it is indeed the "meat" of the Word.[1]

There is far more here than one can glean skimming and scanning. Readers tell us they benefit more by an unhurried and thoughtful examination of this work. Each chapter should be read and "digested" carefully rather than quickly skimmed.

Having satisfied your curiosity, for optimum benefit go back to Chapter One and read through the book chronologically and carefully for overall context and critical knowledge, "line upon line, precept upon precept." This will assure you the highest level of retention and success if you also practice what you learn. In the process of "walking out" your best diet, be certain to listen also to your body, and the Holy Spirit, whose temple we are.

Eatin' After Eden - has dual themes presenting a balance - the positive and the negative. Positively, it presents nutrient-dense healing, sustaining gifts of creative genius; gifts meant for man's enjoyment and benefit since the Fall, and Biblically specified for the latter times as well.

This book also includes several authoritative and riveting[2] chapters identifying and exposing the two chief diets that reject God's plan for eating after Eden. In the long term the "Trojan horse" of the so-called Prudent Diet, and veganism, bring with them enormous consequences for the nation and globally. Profoundly destructive from their conception forward, millions of

---

[1] 1 Cor. 3:14
[2] My four editors described it even more forcefully.

deaths and immeasurable suffering are associated with these. With disability and pain sometimes prolonged for years, millions more may long to die; while others consuming either diet drop dead suddenly with no prior known symptomology. I have known a number of them.

When the Scripture says, "Precious in the sight of the Lord is the death of His saints," it is not referring to these kinds of deaths, whether from deliberate disobedience or lack of knowledge. And whether Christian or non-Christian.[1] Whichever, the consequences are the same. These dietary errors of extremes, are rampant in today's deceived Church. Now *Eatin' After Eden* – teaches a far better way.

Where there is some "overlapping" with a small amount of repetition, certain truths bear repeating for renewing of the mind after so long a time of embedded and ingrained error.

"Christian veganism" is spreading like wildfire in the American church today, a major reason for this work's inclusion of a couple of chapters about this and vegetarianism in general. Having explained the Creator's plan for eating after the Fall, such a book would not be complete without addressing the consequences of rejecting that plan.

Please understand, however, that this book is not about nutrition in general; counterfeit, whole foods, fats, carbohydrates, and phytonutrients, are the subjects of another of a forthcoming work. What *is* presented here is disclosure and information about the Creator's nutrient-dense foods for eating after Eden and the end time. This plan requires animal-source foods as the chief nutrient contributors. This book should convince even the most wary skeptic if they are open to true science and the good Word.

Throughout this treatise you will find abundant scientific references and documentation. Besides that which requires these in a semi-scholarly work and the desire to give credit where credit is due, many readers value them. For those seeking to defame the Creator's power and divine province for our health, they need

---

[1] Though this book may be read by more Christians than non-Christians, nutrition principles are generally applicable to both groups alike.

examine the existing medical literature alone, of which a significant amount is included herein.

A bit of a forewarning is in order. As you seek to enhance your own level of wellness, if you have friends and family yet to realize their responsibility to take care of the bodily temple with which they have been gifted, you may find them irritated and sometimes even irrational about your choice to live proactively. Compare that with the reactive position of lying on an ambulance gurney screaming for help, dependent upon "better living through technology," warns physician Chris Meletis. "Inaction is the active process of choosing to do nothing," as defined by Dr. Meletis.

Take charge, be well, and live proactively! Our Creator wants you enjoying good health, yet He also created us with free will to make personal choices about this. May this well-referenced, scientifically based book reflecting God's plan for eating and wellness, be a blessing to you and yours in helping you and them achieve abundant health for His glory.

1

The Fall: Before & After

Nature's God & Creator

Ordinarily, writers who agree with the Declaration of Independence and that it is a self-evident truth that "...all men are *created*...," nevertheless refer only to Nature rather than the Creator. "Nature" is acceptable to most readers, whether they are Christian or not. Yet that same document also refers to "Nature's God."

The Godhead, *Elohim* (plural), was involved in creating the world, declares Genesis 1:26. Jesus Christ,[1] the Son of God, was the active Creator:[2] "All things were made by Him, and without Him nothing was made that was made," John 1:3 makes clear. Likewise, verses two and ten of Hebrews 1 declare that in the beginning the Son made the worlds and laid the foundation of the earth; the heavens are the works of His hands.

Acting as the Father's agent, it was the Son who actually brought into being the magnificent Eden where He formed and placed the first humans, Adam and Eve.

Little Bit Of Heaven

The first family had perfect environs during their stay in that glorious garden. Some scientists believe a global canopy regulated

---

[1] The spirit of anti-Christ is increasingly manifested in the world today by its hatred of Him, that Name above all names, and those who call themselves by that Name.
[2] Gen.1:1, John 1:1 and1 Cor. 8:6. There are other like Scriptures

humidity, temperature, sunlight and its ultraviolet (UV) rays, air currents, and oxygen mix.[1] Indeed, many fossils of gigantic ferns and tropical animals have been found in what are now frigid areas of the globe, that seem to support that belief.[2] The garden also had "built-in" irrigation. There were no weeds, no briars, no poisonous plants, and no digging or hard labour was required to tend it.

This wondrous divine design of flora and fauna was supported by very rich, deep topsoil essential for superior nutrition. Besides untold numbers of beauteous ornamentals, its edible landscaping thrived with every nutrient that plants require to produce superior nutrients for man and animals. Flawless beings enjoyed faultless digestion, total nutrient absorption, and optimum metabolism. There was perfect health, growth and maintenance for all life.

Perfect love, purity and perfection with total trust between Adam and Eve and in their devoted Father, supported the highest level of intimacy with Him and each other. Growing in the perpetual presence of holy God, they were utterly nourished - spirit, soul, and body. In a word, they experienced *wholeness.*

Mind-boggling Mania

God's first children had it all! Yet they traded the Tree of Life for one piece of forbidden fruit from the Tree of Knowledge of Good and of Evil. This treasonous act resulted in that we know as "the Fall." Dialoguing with the devil didn't work. Standing between them and Almighty God, food became the first idol. The only law pertained to eating and they broke it.

A New & Hostile Environment

Because Adam disobeyed God's first commandment, the ground was cursed for his sake; and in sorrow he ate from it the rest of his life, Scripture reveals. "Therefore the Lord God sent him

---

[1] McLean, Oakland & McLean, *The Bible, Key To Understanding The Early Earth*, 1987

[2] Fossils of coral reefs usually found in warm tropical climates have been found in the Willowa Mountains of Oregon. A baby plesiosaur dinasour fossil was found near the South Pole in 2006.

forth from the Garden of Eden to till the ground from whence he was taken..."

With unaccustomed hard labor, by the sweat of his brow [1] each and every deeply rooted thorn and thistle must be pulled or dug up one at a time.[2] With the newly cursed earth, some plants became toxic. What a rude awakening for poor Adam! He had taken so much for granted...

The Creator planted Adam's first garden before the Fall. The global canopy, dew and mist, with ideal temperatures, helped maintained the friable tilth of the soil when there was no hard, sun-baked earth. But the cursed ground required cultivation with very basic tools of man's own invention.

It was all very stressful. Adam had no experience with this frustrating new life as hard as the resistant soil. There was no John Deere tractor, not even a shovel, or gloves for uncalloused and soon-to-be blistered palms.

Animals who were once submissive, became threatening. Unaccustomed as Adam was to this, he quickly realized the need for substantial shelter to protect his young family, not only from the harsh elements, but from the many previously tame animals turned wild. Yet he had no ready building materials nor carpenter's tools. A cave might well have immediately met that need. Likely many of these animals ate the tender young plants he worked so hard to grow, as soon as the shoots sprang up in his own garden.

At the same time, domestic strife with its stress no doubt sprung up in the uncomfortable home. They wre no longer co-regents.[3] There were also painful childbirth and rebellious children born in sin, adding significant strife. Instead of love, resentment and jealousy were manifested, with one offspring murdering another.

All were exceedingly hard to bear by sinful man. As well, negative thoughts and resentment resulted in toxic emotions. These sins and conditions together, led to diminished digestion,

---

[1] It is assumed that the protective canopy was removed with the Fall.
[2] Eight generations later, Lamech was still still lamenting this, calling his son's name Noah (rest), hoping he would help with the hard toil "...because of the ground which the Lord has cursed." Gen. 5:29
[3] Gen. 1:26-28. Cf. Gen. 3:16 with 4:7.

assimilation and absorption of nourishment. At the same time, far more nutrition was needed for the demands of the harsh, new reality.

Paradise Lost – A New Paradigm

A Christian medical doctor asked what my latest book was about. I replied, "Eatin' after Eden." He responded, "We live by the book **Back To Eden.**" One big problem with that title is denial – man was forever expelled from Eden with its perfect foods. After Adam fell, he soon collided with reality, including that a plant foods diet was *inferior*. It was missing critical nutrients.

Before the Fall, the garden and the perfect body of man, were able to produce total nourishment specific for optimum health. Afterwards, likely man lost the ability to produce the chief macronutrient and other essential ones that the body makes only in part or not at all post-Eden. What we *do* know is that monumental need was beyond the capability of a cursed earth's plants, even thousands of years ago before it "waxed old like a garment;" when its plants offered infinitely higher nutrient levels than today's.

Truly, the Fall ushered in a nourishment deficit that had to be made up if mankind was to continue to the planned end time in which we find ourselves. For this fulfillment, new resources were critical. Thus mankind became dependent upon the Creator in a new way we will explain shortly.

Jehovah Jireh, Our Provider

The Father had been very concerned with His children's diet from the beginning. As parents teach youngsters, even before Eve was taken from Adam's side, He walked and talked with His son and took him on learning tours in the garden. He taught Adam to eat tender greens and the tree fruits which reproduce with seeds.

Even if the foods of Genesis 1:29 could be reproduced today, they lack or are comparatively low in vital substances. Additionally, there are other essential nutrients the body can no longer produce and must obtain from its environment, certain nutrients critical for fallen man long term, especially in the end time.

Quickly, our Provider intervened with His ingenious Nutrition Plan B that has withstood 6,000 years of the most rigorous testing. Several chapters of this book scripturally and scientifically explain and well document that divine provision, specifically crucial not only for ancient man but for us as well. These chapters identify the Creator's unique, most important macronutrients as the core of that marvelous plan - indispensable nutrients millions in and outside the Church are not receiving today due to selective dietary restrictions, the third reason for inadequate nutrition in some groups we will discuss further on in this book.

Divine Nutrition Can Bear Eternal Results

Upon approaching the beginning of the present decade of my life, I asked the Father what He would have me do with it. He responded, "Do the most for the *most*. My people are destroyed for lack of *knowledge*."

I knew I was to spend less time one-on-one with individuals in a counseling practice, and focus on what could also help countless ones, even in far away places, whom I would never meet. Already this book has begun to achieve that.

Yet even if we supply our bodies the best of nutrition, live healthy lifestyles, and though improved quality of life be enjoyed into a ripe old age, we will all eventually die unless our Lord and Savior, Jesus Christ, returns soon. However, there's more to this calling; diet and lifestyle can have *eternal* value.

I have observed that usually sick saints are no threat to the enemy. In order to be more available to God, we need to be as healthy as possible. Prevention of illness is best. The Creator's nutrition is critical for that.

Often physical suffering may be prevented through education such as this book provides. Yet those who become reconciled unto the Father through the ministry of informed, restored ones, and who then teach others that they learn in this book, will avoid the ultimate suffering of eternal separation from God. Best of all, they will enjoy eternal relationship with Him and His family, and they will bear fruit for Him as He commands.[1]

---

[1] True Christianity is not a religion but a relationship of the Father with His children.

A Sidelined Soldier's Restoration

I never shall forget that day I heard someone shouting my name excitedly from the other side of the large restaurant where we were enjoying dinner of fresh, whole-foods. I turned and saw a young man running toward us. Absolutely radiant, Ed quickly introduced himself, and shared this amazing story:

> I attended your seminar at our church a year ago! You didn't know it but I had a brain tumor. Actually, the [state medical school] had already removed three of them, but the last one was inoperable. I was terminal, dying when you came to our church that night.
>
> You explained we should not change our entire diets suddenly. But I went home that night and got rid of everything in my kitchen cabinets. I threw it all in the garbage. The next day I went out and bought *real* food. After three months of eating that, the tumor was gone!
>
> I remembered that you said at the seminar, that we had an obligation to use what we learned, and our increased wellness for God's purposes. I just got back from Mexico, where I shared God's love with many down there who accepted Jesus Christ as their Savior. And I want to thank you so much for coming to our church and teaching us God's truth about His plan for eating today.

No human can cure anyone of anything. We thank God for Ed's obedience to His Word, and this remarkable restoration. Truly, we are "fearfully and wonderfully made."[1] Our Creator designed our bodies to heal themselves in countless ways, twenty-four hours per day. Those in the health care comminity all depend upon that continuing innate drive toward homeostasis.[2] Though Ed's is an unusual case, should we be surprised when restoration

---

[1] Psa. 139:14
[2] The Creator placed within the human body, in each and all of its cells and systems, both the capability and a striving to maintain equilibrium by adjusting physiological processes.

occurs if we stop ingesting toxins and that which inhibits healing, then provide our bodies all that the Great Physician designed for that support,[1] while coming more and more into His will? You will read about other cases in this book, testifying to God's creation's response to that which He designed for its best use.

I am always deeply moved by the love of our Father when He allows me to learn of restored "side-lined soldiers" who return to ministry. Again, it makes my work of 40 years an eternal matter, with eternal rewards for all involved.

All Christians are called to ministry, whether as stay-at-home moms, in the military, as manual laborers or executives – in the church and in the world. There are neighbors, co-workers, service techs, and friends with whom we come in contact who never hear a sermon. We are all called to share God's love and the Gospel of His Son.

It is not by chance but by divine intent that this book came into your hands. You too have an obligation to use its message to help bring increased levels of wellness for the eternal glory of God. You may not be sent to a foreign land as was Ed; yet, there is no greater mission field than America today. May we all be "salt and light," good stewards of His knowledge, good health, and His grace.

---

[1] His nourishment of natural and spiritual foods; exercise, sunlight, fresh air, pure water, proper rest, reduced stress, and fellowship with Him and our fellow man.

2

Eatin' After Eden
With God's Awesome Gifts

Grace Greater Than All Sin

The Father was not taken by surprise when His first children broke His first law. Jehovah Jireh, the Provider, also knew beforehand what they would need - spiritually and naturally - after they transgressed.

"Grace is not only receiving what we *don't* deserve, but receiving it when we deserve something else," it has been said. Though there were unimaginable consequences for all creation, still God loved the disobedient, disloyal pair, and did not abandon them. Among many other things, the Father created for them - and us - that which would provide the most important nutrients this side of the Fall.

Genesis 1:29 Diet: Then And Now

The vegan diet of Genesis 1:29, ideal for man before the Fall, provided vitamins, minerals, trace minerals, phytonutrients,[1] carbohydrates, small amounts of raw fats; and a very small amount

---

[1] Classified differently than protein, carbs, fats, vitamins, and minerals, phytonutrients (phytochemicals) are biologically active nutrients in plants (phyto) that provide their taste, resistance to disease, and color (the darker the color the more beneficial). With approx. 12,000 discovered to date, they help maintain the structure and function of the human body. As well, studies show that various phytonutrients benefit us as antioxidants, anticancer agts., anti-inflammatories, antithrombotics, antibacterials, antivirals, antifungals, cholesterol lowering agts., blood vessel relaxers, immune system stimulants, and intestinal (cont. next p.) bacteria balancers. It pays to eat healthy amounts of dark colored, fresh plant foods.

of protein. That diet lacked adequate amounts of the nutrient critical for *fallen* man, including us today.

Animal-based Foods – God's Special Gifts

Perhaps immediately after the Fall and no later than Genesis 9:3, God commanded man to include flesh foods in his diet. Before you finish reading this book you should understand this as our Father's loving kindness presenting special nutritional gifts to our fallen race, vital for optimum health. We will demonstrate this primary theme by Scripture and nutrition science. Later in this book we will explain animal-based foods (not just flesh foods) as critical in the end time in which we live.

The First Meat Eater: Adam Or Noah?

It was God who first killed animals. In Genesis 3:21 we learn that when Adam and Eve sinned, He took animal skins and made garments for the nearly-nude and no longer innocent pair.[1, 2] Proverbs 27:26 refers to lambs' (skins) for clothing.[3] Probably the Father showed the backsliders how to roast lamb and eat it as would be done later at Passover typifying *the* Lamb yet to come.

Later "...Abel, he **also** brought of the *firstlings* of his *flock*...," Genesis 4:4 tells us. The little adverb "also" lets us know that Adam offered sacrifice as he was taught by the Father. We understand Abel's flock and likely his dad's before him, served for sacrifices, clothing, and food as well, since they would not have

---

[1] This was the beginning of thousands of years of animal sacrifices for Atonement, looking forward to the cross and the true Sacrifice, Jesus Christ our Savior. The lamb Adam's son offered as sacrifice for his sins, typified the Lamb of God who, when He came, would cleanse sin by His blood. By this act, God taught Adam and Eve how terrible sin is, its penalty demanding death after shedding of blood for the remission of sins.

[2] Probably the fig leaf "clothes" didn't last an hour. The pair must have looked utterly rediculous! Had it not been for the somber event, no doubt the Father would have been roaring with laughter watching the two trying to keep the itchy, easily torn leaves over themselves. As it was, perhaps He just shook His head and wept at man's futile effort to cover sin...

[3] See also Heb. 11:37

need for an entire flock for clothing and annual sacrifices.[1] The first food after the Fall was very likely animal-based, complete protein containing fat. Henceforth, that food would provide increased amounts of certain vital nutrients absent in Eden.

Many believe that man was a vegetarian from Genesis 1:29 until 9:3 when Noah was told to eat flesh foods. However, the example of Abel's flock, loss of a global canopy/greenhouse climate, and perhaps other, would seem to discount that.

From the above, it seems eating meat began before Noah left the ark. He knew about clean and unclean animals before the flood, chiefly because man needed the additional nutrition after the Fall. The six extra pair of clean animals Noah took on the ark with him would be needed to produce food for man as well as later sacrifices for Jehovah.

If you choose Genesis 9:3 as the time when meat-eating began, the progression of dietary increase would be Genesis 1:29: vegan diet of tender green plants and fruits; Genesis 3:18: the addition of grains and bread; and Genesis 9:3: the inclusion of flesh foods. Very likely dairy and eggs began before that and provided Noah's family complete protein and fats on the ark.

The exact time that meat eating began, is not critical to know. The important fact is that after the Fall, God commanded man to eat animal-based foods. In so doing, merciful and gracious Father added uniquely signficant nutrition to man's diet, thereby meeting the demands for a tough, new life in a harsh new world. We will examine other Scriptures about this later.

Other Animal-Source Foods

Quality protein comes from animal-source or animal-based foods. Ideally, these are grass-fed, either farm or wild game; eggs from pastured hens, as well as certain fish. Additionally are milk, butter, cream, cheese, yogurt, and kefir, if not ultrapasteurized. They are nutrient-rich foods the Creator added for humans after Eden.

There is a great deal about animal-source foods in the Bible, and hence in this book about God's plan for eating after the Fall.

---

[1] Prov. 27:27 is a similar passage regarding utilitarian goat flocks.

The flesh food of the Bible was only and always organic and grass-fed, whether domestic or wild. Only grass-fed animals convert plant betacarotene to provide antioxidant, real vitamin A (retinol) in liver and dairy products, plus other fat soluble vitamins D, E, and K.

Like the first fallen pair, we too do not enjoy optimum health without adequate amounts of fat-soluble activators animal-based foods contain. These activators are fat soluble vitamins[1] A and D, plus what Dr. Weston A. Price called Activator X, as found in sea foods such as fish liver and roe [fish eggs], butterfat and organ meats from animals feeding on rapidly growing green grass; and to a lesser amount in eggs from pastured chickens.

A common mistake of most patients with serious medical problems, is to believe that "[a] modest amount of high-quality animal foods is enough," says one natural physician.[2] Of course there are exceptions, however, often "more is better" when it comes to these nutrient-dense foods for support of the body and its healing itself, explains Dr. Schmid.

J. R. Crewe, MD, of the Mayo Foundation, forerunner of the Mayo Clinic, Rochester, MN, for 15 years treated many kinds of diseases ranging from cardiovascular (CVD) to tuberculosis. He employed certain detoxification, and certified raw milk as the only food, while obtaining "uniformly excellent" results.[3]

God's Blessing On His Nutritional Gift To Man

Deuteronomy 12:15 and Psalm 107:38, 43 describe meat as a blessing from God. The latter also tells us that a steady supply of meat in the diet is important for fertility and fruitful reproduction: "He blessed them also, so that they are multiplied greatly; and suffers not their cattle to decrease," it declares. Leviticus 11 provides us with a specific list and guidelines for God's sanctified flesh foods of meat, poultry, fish, and even a few insects (remember John the Baptist's locusts!). New Testament Scriptures are included as well in God's dietary instructions and commands.

---

[1] Fat soluble vitamins require fat for absorption.
[2] Schmid, R, *Diet and Recovery from Chronic Disease,* Wise Traditions magazine, Winter 2004-39-45
[3] http://www.realmilk.com/milkcure.html

Protein's Priceless Uses

Animal-source protein was the main contributor to muscles fallen Adam suddenly became aware of with his new strenuous tasks. A strong body was needed for building shelters, handling animals, and tilling the ground. Adequate quality protein was also essential for childbearing by Eve, the mother of us all.

The only substance our bodies have more of than protein is water. Hair, nails, and tissues – all require protein as their "raw material" for building and growth.

Not only is the protein collagen important for bones, it is the main component of soft tissue cartilage, ligaments, and tendons. Of 25 types, it supports our internal organs as well.

Muscle is also essentially protein; without adequate quality protein intake and good digestion, we lose muscle. The body turns to muscle catabolism for protein when it hasn't enough, whether due to poor digestion or inadequate protein intake. You don't want that to happen!

The various systems of the body all function by enzymes and hormones. Protein is required for these, thousands of bodily functions, transport of molecules, blood clotting, growth, heat and energy; for building of new tissues and repair of injured ones; for reproduction, mental health, cell receptors that bind chemicals to assist in their uptake into the cell (e.g., insulin and glucose); and a strong immune system. Immune deficiency is chiefly associated with protein malnutrition.

Some of these internal tasks may have been less critical in the previous sanctuary, but outside Eden's optimal environment, they soon became of vital importance for survival.

What If The Worker Numbers Decreased?

Nothing could happen in our bodies without enzyme "workers." Without them, we could not blink an eye, lift a finger, or digest food. There are digestive enzymes and systemic enzymes. A deficiency can have broad-reaching effects; quality protein is critical for these indispensables.

Then What Is Protein?

The word *protein* comes from the French and Greek, meaning of first or primary importance. Lack of this macronutrient, whether due to maldigestion or dietary insufficiency, leads to premature aging, the opposite of growth. Complete protein is vital for every kind of growth our bodies experience. Healing of free radical damage in tissues requires it. Without quality protein, "fallen man falters."

Complete proteins are complex molecules made up of twenty-two amino acids (A/A). Amino acids are "building blocks" of the body. As end products of protein digestion, they pass through the intestinal wall. From general circulation, each tissue and organ absorbs the specific amino acid it needs to produce its own protein. Patricia Bragg, ND, says, "They are what makes our food turn into us," as they literally become part of our tissue, building muscle, organs and tissues, while circulating in the blood.[1] "The life is in the blood," Scripture informs us.

Nine A/A acids are *essential* in the diet; they cannot be produced in the body today, and likely not since the Fall. The other thirteen are produced in the human liver. All twenty-two *were* likely produced by the body while Adam and Eve enjoyed the Genesis 1:29 diet. Soy is the only plant source of complete protein today. We will discuss that at length in Chapter 7.

This is not to say there were no complete protein foods before the Fall. In fact, unless Adam and Eve's bodies had produced the amino acids for this, plants must surely would have done so.

Basically there is plant protein containing some of the amino acids; and quality protein found only in animal-based foods. The green plants and fruit specified in Genesis 1:29, about which we will have more to say, were not likely high in protein of any kind, and surely not complete protein.

In this regard, before discussing protein further in the next chapter, it is interesting and appropriate to mention a very special kind of fruit that Adam might well have enjoyed before being evicted from the garden.

---

[1] Bragg, P, *Bragg News-Gram,* 2006

Avocado – Another Divine Provision

Today, avocados are native to North America,[1] and are not included in the Bible as such, however, there may have been similar foods in Eden. It is unusual today for fruit to contain protein, however, the likes of it probably grew in the Garden with that paradisiacal climate.

Avocado is extremely high in potassium, 1,300 mg. for Florida avocados and 1,800 mg. for the California fruit. Though other fruits contain chiefly carbohydrates, some vitamins, minerals, and phytonutrients, the amazing avocado also provides a very small amount of the critical *complete* protein. This means it includes all the essential amino acids, as in animal protein. Though it is inadequate for that macronutrient today, it or another such food may have included high amounts in oppulent Eden.

A California student told me that during her financially-strapped college days she ate chiefly avocados she found lying on the ground under trees at various places. That would not provide a meaningful amount of protein, however, she survived and is doing well today.

Yet this unusually nutritious fruit is a source of all macronutrients, including healthy fats, also unusual for fruit. Since it is eaten raw, its enzymes help digest the good fat as well as all the other nutrients in it, including high, provitamin A.

As an Eden-like fruit, this semi-superfood should be enjoyed often for its many nutrients, some fiber, and digestive ease, beginning in early childhood down to the grave. It is an answer to prayer for those unable to chew well.

Be aware that California avocados contain 13 grams of carbs, while Florida ones have a high 27 grams. One half per day is ample for most people.[2]

---

[1] Seeds may have been dispersed during Noah's flood, or carried by explorers or others later.

[2] Interestingly, an extract from avocados looks very promising in the fight against cancer. Tumors thrive on sugar (glucose). This extract, mannoheptulose, prevents glucose uptake by cancers, thereby starving them, with tumor sizes reduced 56-79% in five days in mouse studies. Board, M;

Is Your Body Protein Malnourished?

Amino acid deficiency is often the result of protein deficiency for a number of reasons. The diet may be inadequate; digestion or absorption may be faulty for various reasons including chronic stress, intestinal flora destroyed by antibiotics, or chlorine in the drinking water; food preservatives, and "man-ufactured" foods (foods made by man, not the Creator), which simply are not easily digested.

Infection, trauma, prescription or over-the-counter drugs – all can interfere with protein digestion. There may be imbalances or deficiencies of other nutrients; or age-related issues may be factors. When bioavailable protein is overly reduced for whatever reason, the body may turn to digestion of its own in muscle tissue (catabolism), in order to make up its requirement.

We said that complete protein includes all the EAA. If even one is inadequate or missing from the meal, critical protein synthesis may be impossible. With vegetarianism's popularity today, some have come to believe that all EAA need not be present at the same meal. Why then, would the Creator provide an entire class of complete protein foods that provide all the EAA when eaten?

With so many possible causes for protein and EAA deficiency, it is all the more important to include quality protein that provides all these. Quality protein foods are of first or primary importance.

Complementary Protein

Almost without exception, plant protein lacks adequate amounts of one or more essential amino acids, and is therefore referred to as incomplete protein (we have devoted a full chapter to soy protein). It is possible to obtain complete protein from complementary vegetarian food groups *if* you can remember which

---

Colquhoun, A; Newsholme, E, High Km glucose-phosphorylating (glucokinase) activities in a range of tumor cell lines and inhibition of rates of tumor growth by the specific enzyme inhibitor mannoheptulose. *Cancer Research* (1995) 55, 3278-3285.

foods to combine and how much of each. As you will see in the vegetarian/vegan chapters, very few people are willing or able to devote the amount of time and understanding required for success with this.

Food preparation is also a factor in eating plant foods for complete protein, e.g. cooking beans except at low temperatures renders them carbohydrates rather than good protein sources which require grain for the lysine amino acid.

Because complementary protein provides all the essential A/A does not mean it is a nutritious as animal-sourced protein which has many other nutrients and invaluable properties we will get too shortly.

Meat: Commanded Or Permitted?

A Christian physician asked me whether eating meat is commanded or "just okay." I don't believe God would have added flesh to man's diet, and all that means for humans and animals; or included so much about meat in His Word if eating it is not important for optimum health.[1]

God's directive to Noah in Genesis 9:3 was not a suggestion or option. He was commanded to eat meat given him, the same as tender, green plants from Genesis 1:29. 1 Timothy 4:1-6 addresses this issue specifically for our time as well; we are warned not to reject that which God created and set apart to be eaten with thanksgiving in the last days.

My personal and professional experience with this source of quality protein, is also very convincing for me. However, He has not left us to personal opinion and second guessing. His Word is clear. "What thing soever I command you, observe to do it; thou shalt not add thereto, nor diminish from it," says the Almighty.

---

[1] The term "flesh foods" refers to all animal foods – red meat, poultry, and fish, "meat" refers only to red meats.

Is Genesis 1:29 For Us Today?

Absolutely! Nowhere does Scripture tell us to discontinue eating plant foods. In fact, Genesis 9:3 reaffirms Genesis 1:29 and the value of plants nutritionally:

Every moving thing that lives shall be meat for you; **even as** the green herb have I given you all things.

The Hebrew word for "herb" here is the same as in Genesis 1:29. It is not either/or but *both plants and animals* that our Creator intends for us dietarily today. Each provides different nutritional and other valuable needs. A wide variety of foods from both these groups helps provide balanced nutrition, especially in the end time.

3

Quality Protein – The Best Of The Story!

How Much Do You Need?

Once we understand what the Bible and nutrition science reveal about animal-source quality protein, we must know how best to put it to use for optimum wellness. The first question most ask in this regard, is "How much do I need?"

FDA protein recommended dietary allowance (RDA) is equivalent to 3.6 grams per 10 pounds body weight. Thus, a person weighing 150 pounds would need 54 grams of protein per day according to this agency. This amount may be found in a total of six ounces of flesh food plus a couple of eggs, or plus one egg and eight ounces of milk, per day. Fresh meat, fish, and poultry contain approximately 20% of their weight as complete protein.

One problem with the government's RDA for any nutrient is that it is based upon the need in healthy people.[1] This daily value (DV) represents a minimum to survive, not to thrive.

Neither does this calculation take into account all the growing children, women who are pregnant or nursing, seniors, anyone suffering disability or disease, who is participating in strenuous exercise or hard, manual labor.

---

[1] The government claims "97.5% of the national population are healthy." Is the largest industry in the nation - the sick care industry - for only 2.5% of the population? Why are most Americans terrified of being without health care insurance? Is it that the government doesn't recognize "unhealthy" in its myriad forms? Recall that 70% of all Americans die from heart disease. Go figure…

Other Calculations Of Protein Need

In fact, today's protein needs are calculated in a number of ways. Many nutritionists figure this as a percentage of the total caloric intake per day. Often people find counting calories difficult and a hassle to keep track of; they find it much simpler to control the number of *grams* daily of the nutrients.

Depending upon body fat percentage and generally speaking, the average man may need approximately 70-90 grams of protein each day; women about 10-20 grams less. However, pregnant women may consume 70 grams/day and lactating mothers as much as 80 grams of complete protein. For children the number of grams varies from 25 grams at ages 1-3, to 75 grams/day for young men 14-22 years of age.

We all actually require a certain amount of protein on an ongoing basis. The best we can provide here is a rule of thumb with starting points that will need to be modified sooner or later, depending upon a number of factors, some of which are included in this book.

Science On The Side Of Extra Protein

It may be best to err on the side of a little extra protein since protein (and fats) can be converted in the body for energy as needed. However, glucose and fats cannot be converted to protein.

Several recent studies in the US, Australia, and the Netherlands have shown that a high protein diet not only gives lasting satiety, but a healthy rate of weight loss as well. Australian Manny Noakes, PhD, senior research, finds that "A high-protein meal will sustain people far longer than a high-fat meal or a high-carbohydrate meal."

Additionally, the Netherlands study found that a high protein diet fed at energy balance,[1] compared with just an adequate protein diet, increased not only satiety, but thermogenesis, sleeping metabolic rate (and temperature), protein balance, and fat

---

[1] In biology, energy balance is measured by Energy intake = internal heat produced + external work + energy storage

oxidation. Some health care practitioners are increasing fat as a source of energy, and decreasing carbs.

The Blue Mountains Eye Study performed at the University of Sydney with 2,900 males and females ranging in ages from 49-97, proved that those who consumed the most protein, and vitamins A, B_1, B_2, and B_3 (niacin), "were at lowest risk for developing cataracts."[1] Of course, aging means far less nutrients are absorbed, therefore more are needed to maintain wellness.

If you were an average man, high protein intake might be two eggs and two slices of turkey bacon for breakfast, one large chicken thigh for lunch, and three ounces of cheese on your large green salad for dinner, in order to get your seventy grams of protein in one day. Or you might eat complementary vegetable protein at one meal.

Replacing a diet of refined, highly processed, high carbs with whole-foods, a small amount of complex carbs, quality protein and healthy fats, can help with weight loss and in maintaining an ideal weight.

Words of Caution

Serving as adviser to the nation to improve its health, the Institute of Medicine (IOM) was established in 1970 under the charter of the National Academy of Sciences.[2] The IOM provides independent and objective advice to policymakers, health professionals, the private sector, and the public. Its position is that there is presently no clear evidence that a high protein intake increases the risk of obesity, coronary artery disease, kidney stones, osteoporosis, or cancer.

However, if your body requires eighty grams of protein daily and you eat one hundred-twenty, it may not be able to metabolize the extra protein. The excess must be excreted after liver and kidney processing, which may put a strain on these organs long-term. Whether calcium, protein, or other nutrients, except for short

---

[1] *Opthmology,* 2000; 107:450-456

[2] As a child, my grandfather took me to National Academy of Sciences chapter meetings. I recall one regarding DDT. I still have the notes I took as Walter DeLamer, PhD, spoke about the mosquito problem in the Panama Canal.

periods, very high amounts of intake are usually unhealthy without professional care.

When starving Brazilian children were fed a high protein diet, serious health issues developed until vitamin A retinol was added.

Chronic Stress & Protein Deficiency

Stress prevents good digestion, especially of protein. We have all "learned to live with it," or so we may think. How many consider the stress of simply watching the 6:00 news, or exciting or frightening TV, DVD's, and movies regularly and often while eating dinner?

Actually, it is impossible to live in this "highly developed" nation and avoid many chronic stressors. Add to that, 9-11's whole new level of anxiety for many - chronic fear of the unknown – terror of the terrorists, as well as politicians' and media's handling of the Iraqi war on a daily basis for years. Worry is very stressful.

Nutritional deficiency is another stressor for our bodies. This becomes a vicious cycle since stress itself adds to nutritional requirements. In all these, the protein requirements might be at least another gram or so per day per kilogram of weight, significantly above the RDA recommendation.

We are not "cookie cutter" look alikes, and even in healthy individuals, the amount of nutrient requirement varies from person to person. Ideally you would work with a qualified nutritionist or physician who works with certain testing to determine if your protein intake is adequate. Short of that, you might experiment by increasing or decreasing your intake by 10 grams. A good digestive enzyme formula can also make a difference in how much you require.

The Healthiest Protein Foods

When not overly cooked so as to prevent denaturing of the protein for good digestion and assimilation of the protein, the following list of healthy protein foods provides the number of grams shown (buckwheat and spelt are not high protein foods, however, they are excellent foods with small amounts of good protein):

Protein Food	Number of Grams
2 Eggs[1] (3 g. ea. yolk and egg)	12
2 slices uncured turkey bacon	12
3 oz. ground beef – lightly broiled	21
3 oz. lamb	21
3.5 oz. sauteed chicken	26
3.5 oz. salmon (not overcooked)	27
1 cup of milk or yogurt	8
3.5 oz. buckwheat seed or flour[2]	13
2 oz. spelt (Ex. 9:31, Ezek. 4:9)[3]	10

Some Signs of Protein Deficiency

We've all viewed news footage of "Third World" countries in starvation - close ups of Kwashiorkor, severe protein deficiency. Most of the deficiency in the US is not dramatic and obvious. It is no less real, however. Brittle hair and nails, alopecia, delayed wound healing, muscle weakness and wasting, and low thyroid, are but a few indications of this deficiency. We shall address others as well.

---

[1] Egg white and yolk have 3 g. protein ea. Raw egg white inhibits B vit. biotin's utilization.
[2] Buckwheat is very nourishing with its complete protein, mg., phos., fiber, and many other nutrients.
[3] The same amt. of all purpose white wheat flour contains 2.74 g. of protein.

Protein & Your Blood Sugar Stability

We also need protein for stable blood sugar.[1] Some people experience symptoms of low blood sugar, including becoming shaky and very hungry, craving chocolate, sugar, or other foods, when they are not getting adequate protein. Fatigue is often found with low or low quality protein consumption. Today's high carb breakfasts of little protein can set you up for all the above.

Protein & The Immune System

Weak immunity can be a sign of low protein intake, inadequate stomach acid to digest it even in younger people, or inability to utilize this essential nutrient.[2] We will have more to say about the immune system and protein digestion.

Dem Bones, Dem Bones, Dem Dry Bones...

Most everyone knows about bone's requirement for calcium, but did you know that protein is one of the nutrients essential for healthy bones? Actually, many nutrients are required for bone-building;[3] however, bone matrix requires a great deal of protein for collagen, without which bones crumble.[4] Writes nutritionist Susan Brown, PhD:

> Protein is important to the integrity of bone at all life stages and protein restriction has been shown to limit bone density, reduce growth hormone, and increase both fracture risk and fracture healing time [5]

---

[1] Studies show that higher protein is helpful for Type II diabetes.
[2] There may be other reasons for recurring colds and infections, e.g., high sugar intake, hypothyroidism, *et al.* Quality, adequate protein is important for a healthy thyroid.
[3] See Exhibit A after Chap. Seven for list of these.
[4] Homocysteine is commonly elevated in CVD, and also osteoporosis, interfering with collagen production.
[5] Brown, S., *Bone Health eNewsletter,* Summer 2005

There are many factors involved, however, we know that quality of bone diminishes in the elderly who often cannot chew meat.

Subjects of an Australian study reported in 2005 in the *American Journal of Clinical Nutrition*, involving 1,077 women average age 75, consumed a mean of 80.5 grams of protein/day. The dose-response effect showed that subjects who consumed less than 66 grams of protein per day had significantly lower qualitative ultrasound of the heel and hip than did the subjects who ate more than 87 grams protein/day. The conclusion was that: "These data suggest that protein intakes for elderly women above current recommendations may be necessary to optimize bone mass."[1] Diminished protein digestion capability of the elderly with decreased stomach acid may be a significant factor in longevity.

Are We Promoting An Acidic Diet?

Some nutritionists believe a diet including more than minimal acid-forming protein, may lead to acidosis; causing the body to pull alkaline calcium from the bones, they say. Other health care practitioners hold that except in severe illness, the body balances its pH (acid/alkaline level).

As in Bible times, today alkaline foods such as almonds, apples, asparagus, citrus fruits (alkali-forming after digestion), figs, grapes, melons, olives, onions, parsley, raisins, raw spinach, unheated honey, and dark green leafy vegetables, balance that – *if* eaten regularly. Homemade vegetable broth is an extremely alkalizing agent. Unfortunately, today's Americans eat few fruits and vegetables to compensate for acid-forming protein foods. In Genesis 9:3 our Creator recognizes the need for this balance and commands Noah to include the tender greens of Genesis 1:29 with his meat.

Herta Spencer, MD, found that both animal and human studies that correlated calcium loss with high protein diets, used isolated,

---

[1] Devine, et al, Protein consumption is an important predictor of lower limb bone mass in elderly women, U. of W. Aus, Sir Charles Gardner Hosp, Aus, W. Australian Institute of Med. Rsrch, Perth, Aus, Biomed. & Health Sci. Edith Cowan U. Perth, Aus, & the Sch of Pub. Hlth, Curtin UTech, Perth, Aust, June 2005

fractionated amino acids from milk or eggs.[1] In Dr. Spencer's studies the participants showed *no increase in excreted calcium while eating meat protein, or any significant change at all in serum calcium, even over extended periods.*[2] Other investigators found that a high protein intake actually increased calcium absorption when dietary calcium was adequate and more than 500 mg. per day.[3] (Chocolate, including chocolate milk, contains calcium-binding oxalates, and may interfere with calcium absorption.)

If one engages in an unhealthy lifestyle, with poor diet of high refined carbs, toxic fats, and low calcium intake, plus a lack of many nutrients required for calcium absorption, one might expect potential bone loss as compared with those who are health-conscious, enjoy a whole foods diet, including abundant amounts of quality dairy product. We should not overeat non-protein, acid-forming foods, e.g. grains, rice, bread, and nuts other than almonds.[4]

Easily absorbed, alkalinizing mineral supplements are a must regardless of one's position on acidosis. There are many other important reasons to avail one's self of these foods and supplements.

Check Your Toes!

One interesting sign of amino acid deficiencies as taught by Stu Wheelwright, son of A. S. "Doc" Wheelwright, internationally known herbologist, is that such lack causes vertical lines on the bottoms of the four toe stems to the right and left of the big toe. Jack Tipps, ND, PhD, found these lines lighten and go away within two to eight months as overall health improves.[5] I cannot verify this but it would be interesting if you have such lines, to improve your level of wellness with God's plan for eating after the Fall.

---

[1] Spencer & Kramer, Factors contributing to osteoporosis, *Journal of Nutrition*, 1986 116:316-319

[2] Spencer & Kramer, Further studies of the effect of a high protein diet as meat on calcium metabolism, *Amer. Jnl. of Clncl Nutr*, June 1983 37 (6):924-929

[3] Linkswiler, et al, Calcium retention of young adult males as affected by level of protein and of calcium intake, *Trans. N Y Acad Sci* 1974 36:333

[4] White rice has very little nutrition; the usual brown rice smells rancid. Small amts. of brown Basmati rice are a better choice.

[5] Tipps, J, *The ProVita Plan,* Apple-A-Day Press, TX, 1996

SAMPLE MENU

The following menu provides approximately 60-70 grams of complete protein for one day and comparatively low carbs, with amounts to be adjusted as needed.

Breakfast: Two large eggs over easy in 1 Tbsp. coconut butter. ½ cup whole spelt soaked overnight and simmered in a.m.; or buckwheat (cook only about 10-15 min.), or 1 slice warmed, sprouted grain bread. Two slices turkey bacon. 4 oz. herb tea of choice.

Lunch: *Fiesta Salad*
Layer torn Romaine & raw spinach with chopped red bell pepper, ½ cubed, firm, avocado; ½ cup warm black beans (optional); sprinkle with Tbsp. green pumpkin seeds, 1 oz. shredded raw cheese; add 1 Tbsp. sour cream, then salsa - all from health food store or supermarket organics. Eight oz. glass whole milk, not ultrapasteurized.

Dinner: Chicken and Lentils from recipe at end of this book.

Thyroid & Protein Intake Amounts

Thyroid expert Dr. Broda Barnes found that in general, though adequate quality protein is important for the thyroid, high protein requires high thyroid levels to metabolize, else the biological "furnace is overly dampered" as I like to explain it.[1] Arbitrarily significantly increasing protein may not be wise without knowing your thyroid health.[2] On the other hand, hyperthyroidism and

---

[1] Barnes & Galton, *Hypothyroidism, The Unsuspected Illness,* Harper & Row, 1976:155-195

[2] A qualified practitioner should be consulted in determining the proper amount of protein in cases of thyroid dysfunction.

higher levels of thyroid hormone may require more protein for the higher metabolism.

A physician who understands that sub-clinical (not evidenced by tests results) thyroid conditions are just as real, can be very beneficial, according to Dr. Barnes. The issue may be in the tissue; i.e., how well the T4 hormone is converted to the usable T3 form.[1]

Digestion of Protein

Without adequate protein for digestive enzymes and absorption, cellular toxification and starvation will eventually occur. Thus good health is closely associated with good protein digestion.

You may have heard the saying, "You are what you eat." More accurately, you are what you eat, digest, and assimilate! 'Even the most nutrient-dense, properly prepared, organic foods are worse than useless if not well digested.

If protein sits in the stomach too long due to low stomach acid (hypohchlorhydria), then moves on without adequate digestion, it becomes a source of toxins rather than nourishment. A good digestive enzyme formula may save the body's enzyme bank. A qualified practitioner is important for help with the appropriate formula selection.

Some complementary[2] physicians perform the Heidelberg test or use Gastrocaps to detect low hydrochlorich acid (HCl), the most accurate diagnosis. In days past, country doctors used to advise patients to drink a teaspoon of raw apple cider vinegar in a glass of water with their meals. If it burned they were said to have too much stomach acid and they shouldn't take it. If it didn't burn, they were considered to have low hydrochloric acid and needed that much and possibly more.[3] We enjoy organic raw apple cider vinegar with extra virgin olive oil for salad dressing as well.

---

[1] http://www.wilsonssyndrome.com/ is a good laymen's source of info regarding the "tissue issue."

[2] Complementary physicians, usually MDs, employ both medical and alternative modalities in their practices.

[3] Hydrochloric acid also destroys bad bacteria, parasites and yeasts. A lack of it may lead to GI infection, food allergy, autoimmune and degenerative diseases. Don't guess, consult a qualified physician.

Another easy test used to determine normal stomach acid was to take one-quarter teaspoon of baking soda in eight ounces cool water upon arising in the morning. Normally one should burp within two or three minutes, no more than five minutes. Very early, repeated burping was said to mean excessive stomach acid. However, self-diagnosing and "prescribing" in these cases is not advisable. A good complementary or naturopathic physician (ND) will get to the root cause if there is either too much or too little HCl.

Real Salt & Protein

The Bible speaks of salt; but what has salt to do with protein and flesh foods? It is vital to stomach digestion. The production of adequate stomach acid requires real salt. Here again, we must differentiate between altered and God-given nutrients. America's typical diet consists of processed foods high in altered sodium and low in potassium-rich fresh foods.

Is It Your Salt Shaker?

The salt content of food is only about ten percent. Consumers add another five to ten percent total salt intake when eating. A whopping seventy-five percent of sodium in US diets is derived from processed foods, added by the manufacturers and restaurants before you ever pick up your fork!

Excess of inorganic sodium is not due entirely to sodium in table salt, though there are good reasons not to use supermarket salt. Such sodium is not only used in processed foods as sodium chloride, but concealed in food additives such as sodium benzoate saccharin, monosodium glutamate (MSG), and sodium nitrate.

Sodium nitrates are found in nearly all processed, packaged meats, from deli lunch meats to bacon. In the gut they may be converted to nitrosamines, cancer-causing substances. These and thousands of other processed foods are chief sources of excess and unhealthy sodium. Too much of it may lead to a sodium/potassium imbalance. Consuming a diet of all fresh foods avoids it.

Interestingly, some studies and an analysis of data from a preliminary prospective study of patients with confirmed, advanced atherosclertoic CVD, found that "fasting insulin rather than salt is the major driver of hypertension." James H. Hayes, MD, reported the finding at the annual conference of the American Association of Clinical Endocrinologist in June (AACE), 2006.[1]

Mineralized, real salt from the health food store, salt that has not been heated to high temperatures, has no anticaking agents, aluminum, and sugar, is clearly the healthiest. Balancing potassium is found in high amounts in fresh fruits and vegetables such as avocados, raw spinach[2], beet greens, fresh figs, melons, and nectarines (bananas are high in sugar). Milk and yogurt also contain good amounts.

Nimble Joints

Dr. Bernard Jensen found that often when there are digestive[3] or joint problems, there is *low* blood sodium. This nutrient is that which made his Nubian goats so nimble, said he. Following his own teaching, this Christian health care practitioner, lived well into his nineties.

In Dr. Jensen's book, *Goat Milk Magic*, he addresses the issue of "man-ufactured" versus God-made sodium.[4] Real sodium in the bloodstream helps maintain calcium in solution. It is essential for proper balance of fluids, transmission of nerve impulses, acid/alkaline balance, osmotic pressure of cell membrane, and muscle contraction. In fact, sodium is stored in the stomach, walls, bowel, and joints.

Just as the thyroid and other parts of our bodies require organic iodine, so too the adrenal glands (stress glands) require organic sodium. Celery, squash, zuchini and certain sea salt from the health food store, are good sources of natural sodium for the adrenals.

---

[1] Peck P, *MedPage Today*, June 28, 2006
[2] Cooked spinach has toxic oxylates. See Norman Walker, DSc, *Fresh Vegetable & Fruit Juices,* pp. 62, 63.
[3] Recall that sodium is required for stomach acid to digest protein.
[4] Jensen, B, *Goat Milk Magic,* 1994-60

Protein Malnutrition In Surgical Patients

Young and old alike today suffer malnutrition as the result of the Standard American Diet (SAD). In surgical patients, malnutrition is the chief variable associated with slow/poor healing, high rate of complications, morbidity (disease), and mortality (death). This induced suppression of the immune system may include progressive weight loss, weakness, and infections.

The most severe malnutrition issues in hospital settings are associated with protein. Proteins and their amino acids have almost no storage in the body, thus malnutrition first affects them. Such deficiency directly impairs organ function and the immune system with its dependence on protein interaction.

Albumin, The Transporting Protein

Substances are not simply dumped in the blood, they require carriers to transport them. Serum albumin, as an important transporting protein for nutrients,[1] hormones, drugs, and toxins, is synthesized by the liver from adequate dietary protein. Involved in more than sixty-five biological functions, it is said that the higher the serum albumin, the fewer cancers and heart attacks.

A study reported in the *Journal of the American Medical Association* (JAMA) of 54,215 major, noncardiac surgical cases, was undertaken to determine the most reliable predictor of surgical morbidity and mortality. Of the myriad considered, preoperative serum albumin levels proved to be the greatest predictor.[2] This test "...should be used more frequently as a prognostic tool to detect malnutrition and risk of adverse surgical outcomes...," was the conclusion reached by the nutrition scientists and medics who conducted the study and thirty day follow-ups. The study further freported:

---

[1] Lipoproteins transport fat, cholesterol, and other fat-soluble molecules.
[2] Gibbs *et al,* Preoperative Serum Albumin Level as a Predictor of Operative Mortality and Morbidity: National VA Surgical Risk Study, *JAMA*, Arch Surg 1999; 134: 36-42.

Epidemiological studies have demonstrated that low albumin levels [less than 4 mg./dL] are associated with an increased risk for mortality from both cardiovascular (CVD) disease and cancer, whereas life expectancy is highest at high-normal albumin levels. Low albumin may be serving as a marker for other pathogenic processes or factors - infection, inflammation, loss of lean mass associated with illness, undernutrition or lack of activity - but may also reflect a serum antioxidant deficit that contributes to risk.

The most accurate evidences of malnutrition and failing health in surgical and elderly patients are low albumin (hypoalbuminemia), and low cholesterol (hypocholesterolemia). [1,2]

Chris Meletis, ND, recipient of the 2003 Naturopathic Physician Award by the American Association of Natural Physicians, finds that albumin production is dependent not only upon protein but also upon overall metabolic rate. Since metabolism is associated with thyroid, albumin should increase with thyroid improvement.

Healing of all kinds requires quality protein. Muscles undergo tear down if you work out. Adequate protein is essential for that rebuilding as well as all damaged tissue. Family members who were surgical patients healed incredibly fast when they drank pre- and post-op nutrient-dense smoothies high in easily digested quality protein and other nutrients as contained in raw egg yolks and raw goat milk as soon as digestion returned.[3]

---

[1] Sullivan DH, Wall RC, Lipschitz DA. Protein-energy undernutrition and the risk of mortality within 1 yr. of hospital discharge in a select population of geriatric rehabilitation patients. Am J Clin Nutr 1991;53:599-605; Verdery RB, Goldberg AP. Hypocholesterolemia as a predictor of death: a prospective study of 224 nursing home residents. J Gerontol 1991;46:M84-90.

[2] Hypocholesterolemia as a predictor of death: a prospective study of 224 nursing home residents. J Gerontol 1991;46:M84-90.

[3] Patients should check with their doctors when changing their diets.

The Simple Test

Though used in diagnosing and monitoring treatment of a number of diseases and conditions, albumin is a fair indication of general health and nutrition. A single, inexpensive serum albumin test may be useful to confirm adequate quality protein intake and absorption. I like to see my blood albumin not less than 4.5 g/dL.

Albumin is made by the liver and excreted by the kidneys, hence a physician may also order the serum test when there is liver or kidney disease. Or when serum albumin is low, physicians may check for poor liver function. It is also included as part of a comprehensive metabolic panel (blood chemistry) for wellness checks.

Maintaining Your Blood Albumin Level

As we have shown, protein is critical to maintaining a healthy albumin level. Just as the body steals calcium from the bones to maintain a constant blood level of that mineral, so too it strives to keep the serum level of albumin stable.

When there is inadequate protein intake/assimilation, the body turns again to muscle to obtain sufficient amino acids for its synthesis of serum albumin. If the transporter albumin is low, even the highest quality food will not be made available to the cells.

Limiting meal fluids to no more than four ounces,[1] increasing quality protein, and taking digestive enzymes, may help enhance albumin levels. Adequate water, zinc and selenium intakes may also be helpful.

How Often Did The Ancients Eat Meat?

We are not told in Scripture exactly how often meat was eaten. However, certain texts are revealing.

> ...And the Lord appeared unto [Abraham]...in the heat of the day...and [he] said, "My Lord, if now I have

---

[1] Probably most people use mealtime liquids to wash their food down rather than chewing it 30 times each bite.

found favor in thy sight, pass not away, I pray thee from thy servant:...And I will fetch a morsel of bread..." And Abraham ran into the herd, and fetched a calf tender and good, and gave it unto a young man; and he hasted to dress it. And he took [bread,] butter and milk, and the calf which he had dressed, and set it before them...[1, 2]

Here we have three animal-source foods served at a meal as fitting for the Lord himself. Have you noticed there always seemed to be a fatted calf in the ancient times of the Bible? Veal is very nutritious. We all know the story of the Prodigal Son's return in Luke 15 and the ecstatic father. A large celebration was called for and the father told the servants: "...bring here the fatted calf and kill it, and let us eat and be merry."

Then there's the story of Gideon who, when the Angel of the Lord came to visit him, said to Him:

...If now I have found favor in Your sight, then show me a sign that it is You who is talking with me. Do not depart from here, I pray, until I come to You and bring out my offering and set it before You." And He said, I will wait until you return." [3]

So Gideon prepared a kid (young goat), unleavened flour cakes,[4] and broth. Here we see the custom of offering meat to even unexpected callers.

There was no refrigeration, and we have no record that flesh foods were dried in Bible times. Exodus 12:9 instructs Israel not to keep meat overnight. It would require more than one family to butcher and eat a large animal. But highly nutritious small animals such as calves, lambs, goats, fish, poultry, and others were quickly butchered, cooked, and eaten the same afternoon.

---

[1] Gen. 18:6-8

[2] Gal. 3:14 tells us that the blessing of Abraham comes upon believing Gentiles through Jesus Christ.

[3] Judges 6:19

[4] Perhaps the unleavened bread rather than the usual sourdough, was offered to save time.

There are exceptions; however, unless one is fasting, usually one should consume quality protein daily. They might easily have been eaten daily since the Israelites had large flocks and herds of sheep, cattle, and goats according to many Scriptures. Dairy products and even eggs were likely daily fare as well. The New Testament speaks of meat markets in nations where Paul evangelized and planted churches; smaller cuts could be purchased daily even as today in many countries.

Deuteronomy 14:27-29 specifically commands God's people in the principle of providing meat for spiritual leaders who have no land on which to raise meat animals; as well for widows, orphans, and strangers, in order that "...the Lord may bless thee in all the work of thine hand which thou doest." Earlier in that same text, Scripture gave instructions concerning another special occasion regarding eating meat from large animals. Since large animals were not eaten daily, that meat was *greatly* enjoyed on special days, that passage discloses.

Eskimos Without Carbs

The Canadian Eskimos' diet formerly consisted almost entirely of animal foods such as fish, wild meat, and raw whale blubber. Except for a few berries preserved in whale oil, their diet contained essentially no carbohydrates.

The nutrition pioneer, Icelander physician and anthropologist Dr. Vilhjalmur Stefansson spent fifteen years among these Eskimos. Completely adapting himself to that lifestyle and diet, this medic and scientist observed these primitives suffered none of our modern day "plagues" of high blood pressure, coronaries, cancers, strokes, diabetes, and especially obesity. They died at a ripe old age, as did many in recorded Scripture.

The lack of obesity amazed the good doctor because they consumed huge amounts of fatty foods with high calories that surely would have resulted in this *had the foods been of carbs,* proving that "a calorie is a calorie" is untrue!

Furthermore and equally amazing when contrasted with today's myriad obstetric and gynecological complaints, the Eskimo women suffered no such, including no complicated, difficult pregnancies, births, or breast feeding problems. Their mental and emotional stability was free of the high level of social problems of our day. They were a happy people, Dr. Stefansson observed.

Not until about 1900 when these natives were reached with "civilized" peoples' high carbohydrate foods, did all this change for the worse. Also like Weston A. Price, Stefansson noted that tragically, those civilizations that switch to western refined foods, develop all the western diseases that are responsible for building western medicine into the most powerful and wealthy industry in America, if not the entire world.

As an anthropologist Stefansson was first to note it was not the racial origins of Eskimos as scientists had always held, but the ancient nutritional form that protected them from western-type diseases. In fact, some other people groups still exist almost entirely upon animal-based foods even today.

These nutrition pioneers and others proved that there has never been a society that existed without adequate dietary animal-based foods, be they real kefir, soured milk, or other raw dairy products; livestock, wild meat, birds, insects, or various others.

We must also not omit the other important health factors of exercise, fresh air, water, sunshine, adequate sleep, and absence of the powerful stressors of our highly developed society, including the stress of cellular starvation.

Let's not forget the Creator himself grew the organic, wild animal foods on which Eskimos and so many other people groups thrived.

The Proof In Stefansson's Meat "Pudding"

Soon after Dr. Stefansson's remarkable discoveries and exposure of unhealthy, money-making food products, "junk science" set about "debunking" real nutrition science, and the slander-slinging was anything but positive. He was blatantly accused of fabricating the entire report that deflated prideful professionals on their pedestals.

To prove his integrity and the validity of his findings - that the conclusions were more than theories - the bold and brave Dr. Stefansson and Karsten Anderson who had traveled with him in the frigid regions, chose to "risk their lives" as it was thought by the day's medical community, with an unheard of experiment. Under the watchful eye and supervision of New York's Bellevue Hospital, they submitted to the then famous metabolic expert, Eugene Dubois.

Anderson had been healthy as a horse while accompanying Stefansson but since his return to Florida, and eating a high carb diet, he was constantly ill. In 1928 they were admitted to Bellevue and began the diet of fresh, raw, meat only. They ate nothing else but meat. After an entire year, there were no signs of any nutritional deficiency, including vitamin C.[1] Anderson also "felt extraordinarily well," lost excess poundage, and chronic issues that had bothered him previously also "dropped off." Dubois' final commentary was that "the most remarkable thing about the experiment was that nothing remarkable occurred."

Later, Dr. Stefansson's widow wrote Wolfgang Lutz, MD, that her husband had returned to his "friendly Artic diet" and had continued it until his death, convinced of its value not only for weight loss, but also disease prevention, including heart disease.

Many years later Atkins took up from there with his diet of low carbs, high fats, and high amounts of flesh foods. However, that diet varies, particularly its packaged, processed foods, with some of those ingredients.

Tragically, in a nation becoming sicker by the day, relatively few know of these and other nutrition pioneers' work and remarkable discoveries essential for optimum health. We may find we need different proportions of the macronutrients than others, but adequate amounts of each are essential, especially quality protein.

A high carb, low-fat diet may exhaust the pancreas and its production of insulin, and prevent emptying of the gallbladder so as to lead to stone formation.[2]

Word Of Caution

We include Dr. Stefansson's experiment to make a point. It worked well for him and he returned to it later in life for health's

---

[1] Raw and rare meat contains vit. C complex
[2] Gallbladder health may also include avoiding *unhealthy* fats such as highly processed vegetable oils and partially hydrogenated, altered fats (transfats).

sake. However, this is not a balanced diet that would necessarily work for everyone. Dr. Stefansson was a researcher and physician with many years experience with this diet. It is not to be undertaken without professional, qualified monitoring.

Scripture tells us we should cook our meat, howbeit healthfully. The Eskimos ate raw animal-based foods perhaps for convenience. However, raw meat, poultry and fish may contain pathogens and parasites that can make some people very ill. I opened a thawed package of fish and watched in horror as a large ascarid (round worm) crawled out.

Some people may have conditions preventing easy conversion of fats and protein to energy. Especially would such an experiment be inadvisable without clean, organically grown and/or wild meats. And certainly those with liver or kidney diseases should not try it.

Major diet changes, even good ones, usually should not be made suddenly, e.g., moving from a high carb, low protein, low fat diet to a much higher protein, high fat, low carb regimen.

Moderation, Not Gluttony

In Proverbs 30:8, the wise man prays for his allotted daily bread, rather than too much at one time.[1] Proverbs 23:19-21 counsels us as follows:

> Hear thou my son and be wise; and guide thine heart in the way. Be not among winebibbers, among riotous eaters of flesh; for the drunkard and the glutton will come to poverty...

Christians are now considered to be the largest group of obese people in the US. Our potlucks, ice cream socials, after church meals, and plain gluttony are showing. However, it isn't meat chiefly that is our undoing but bar-b-que and deep fried foods, together with refined carbs.

---

[1] "Convenient" as the KJV has it here, is one translation of the Hebrew *kokhe*. However, the context of Prov. 30:8 has to do with temperance, gluttony, and allotted daily bread as Jesus referred to in the Lord's Prayer.

The Hebrew translated here as "riotous" by the King James, can have a number of meanings, however, the same word is translated "glutton" in the next verse. This Scripture is not telling us not to eat meat, which would be contrary to many other passages, but to eat moderately, even as we are to eat everything else. "Hast thou found honey? Eat only so much as is sufficient for thee!" [1]

Meatless Sabbath?

Since meat was not dried overnight in Bible times,[2] and there were to be no fires built on Sabbath, it would seem to be a meatless day. There would have been milk, yogurt, butter, sourdough bread, nuts, fresh and dried fruits and vegetables, and other foods that don't require cooking. Mama and servants got the day off.

Indeed, one meatless day each week may be a healthy practice today as well. I have included a recipe in the back of this book for that purpose, supplying good complete protein and complex carbs.

---

[1] Prov. 25:16
[2] Cooked meat and other leftovers kept more than a day even under refrigeration, may acquire molds.

4

America's Rejection Of God's Nutrition Plan

PART I

There is a way that seems right unto man, but the end there of are the ways of death.[1]

"Thou shalt not surely die…"

Beginning with Eden, the Deceiver, who "comes to kill, steal, and to destroy," has plied his trade.[2] Eve was the first human deceived.[3] She then rejected God's Tree of Life for the Tree of Knowledge of Good and of Evil, a mixture.

The enemy's modern dietary deception, his weapon of mass destruction (WMD), is likewise a mixture. Here you will learn about the so-called Prudent Diet that was ironically conceived of and presented to the nation through one of the most highly respected and trusted health organizations.

Still embraced by physicians, conventional nutritionists, public health authorities, and particularly those concerned with cardiovascular disease (CVD), this "WMD" sprang from the flawed lipid hypothesis. That theory, which follows, will surely be familiar to you as to hundreds of millions since 1956.

---

[1] Prov. 14:12
[2] John 10:10
[3] Adam was not deceived, he knowingly disobeyed God's command to him. (Gen. 3:13, Rom. 5;14, 1 Tim. 2:14) The Creator became the Redeemer of them both.

Saturated Fat: The Heart's Greatest Enemy?

According to the lipid hypothesis,

> Saturated fat increases blood cholesterol, which causes arterial fatty plaque, leading to atherosclerosis, heart disease, and myocardial infarction [heart attack from a clot obstructing a coronary artery].

Like evolution, it appears this theory too assumes facts not in evidence. Yet the unimaginable consequences of acting upon it as fact, have accrued not only to America, but to much of the world.[1]

This assumption was posited by Ancel Keys, PhD in the fifties. Low-fat guru, Nathan Pritikin, MD, was the best known proponent of the theory. Key's controversial Seven Country Study presumed a strong association between cardiovascular disease (CVD[2]) and the amounts of dietary saturated fat and cholesterol.[3] He was accused of having been selective in the countries he used for his study, ignoring those not useful for his conclusion.

Keys' study was questioned by many other studies receiving far less publicity than those funded and supported by the food oil industry. Later in this chapter we will discuss his recommended diet in more detail since its principles still govern most Americans' food choices. It is noteworthy that Keys himself turned to the Mediterranean diet later.

"The Greatest Health Scam Of The Century"

George V. Mann, ScD, MD, involved with the famous Framingham Heart Study and extensive studies of the Maasai, observed in study participants "very high saturated fat intake, atherosclerosis [normal aging], but no coronary heart disease [CHD] at all." Fifteen years ago, this scientist/researcher warned:

---

[1] It is not within the scope of this book to discuss the subject at length, however, Uffe Ravnskov, MD, PhD, and a host of others have authored comprehensive works explaining the scientific truth about saturated fats and cholesterol. See Resources at the end of this book.

[2] CVD is a group of conditions and diseases, all having to do with the heart and/or blood vessels.

[3] *Lancet*, 1957;i:959

The diet-heart hypothesis has been repeatedly shown to be wrong, and yet, for complicated reasons of **pride, profit, and prejudice,** the [lipid] hypothesis continues to be exploited by scientists, fund-raising enterprises, food companies and even governmental agencies. The public is being **deceived** by the greatest health scam of the century.[1]

Man's "New & Improved" Nutrition Plan

Built upon the foundation of the unproven lipid hypothesis, the Prudent Diet's first and primary problem is that *it rejects God's plan for eating after the Fall,* particularly a significant part of His animal-based foods. The PD is high in polyunsaturated vegetable oil.

Though few today know it by that name, you will come to recognize this fifty year old blunder as an example of man's wisdom and logic at their worst.

Since a traditional diet did not cause CVD for eons, when these diseases began to appear, wouldn't it have made sense to ask what had been changed, added, or removed that might cause them? What had been added was *not* saturated fat!

Yet for the masses saturated fat is to be avoided at all cost. For generations they have been taught a strong but groundless aversion to an important part of a healthy diet, and that which the human body requires for a number of important reasons. Wrote one government health official:

> [It is] the belief that total dietary fat and saturated fat [are] primary dietary determinants of serum total and low-density lipoprotein (LDL) cholesterol levels, not dietary cholesterol. Hence…health authorities focus…on **reducing saturated fat and trans fats** in the…diet to help lower blood cholesterol levels rather than focusing on limiting dietary cholesterol.[2]

---

[1] Mann GV, Coronary Heart Disease – Dietary Sense & Nonsense, *Veritas Soc,* London, 1993

[2] McDonald B, The Canadian Experience: Why Canada Decided Against an

Practically parroting Keys, a leader of the "anti-cholesterol army," this official is saying that dietary fat, specifically saturated and trans fat,[1] not dietary cholesterol, are the primary cause of serum total cholesterol and "bad" cholesterol. It is interesting that saturated fat is isolated in that statement, from "total dietary fat." Also, that "saturated and trans fats" are coupled and both recommended for reduction though many studies show they affect serum lipids (blood fats) very differently.

So Great A Loss

Rather than urging return to the proven traditional diet when there was no CVD, the PD officially pronounced "healthy" the addition of now-known toxic, diminished-nutrient foods found increasingly in America's diet since the invention of industrialized foods. The hardest working muscle in the body, the heart requires constant nourishment and properties that red meat and dairy products provide. Touting highly processed vegetable oils plus hydrogenated vegetable oil, the PD also sanctioned denigrating and removal of critical whole foods, without awareness of the loss of their coronary protection and support.

Saturated Fat: More Than Optional

There are a number of other very important reasons to consume animal-source saturated fats.[2] The body uses them for

- Hormone production
- Cell signaling, e.g., adrenaline for "flight or fight" *et al*
- Cell membrane
- Age related loss of white blood cell function
- Tumor prevention

Upper Limit for Cholesterol, Jnl of the Amer Coll of Nutr, Vol. 23, No. 90006, 616S-620S (2004)

[1] These two are regularly linked together in conventional literature.

[2] The Weston A. Price Foundation provides extensive information at its website regarding these.

In fact, there are many benefits from saturated fats.[1] It is found in meat, butter (its butyric acid helps good bacteria adhere to the intestinal lining); breast milk (its lauric acid, found chiefly in coconut butter and palm oil, acts as an antimicrobial); palm oil (its palmitic acid is very important for our lungs); and dairy products.

Degenerative diseases have become rampant since this ailing nation turned to the PD increasingly, to avoid saturated fats. Yet more than half the fat in beef is monosaturated fat, the same as heart-healthy olive oil. Only about one-sixth of beef's saturated fat may raise cholesterol in some people. In fact, based upon the USDA composit data, a three ounce serving of red meat has only a minimal 1.5 grams more saturated fat than the same weight in skinless chicken. The data have become important – only because of the misinformation regarding animal saturated fat.[2]

MI's & The Murderous Truth!

The World Health Organization's (WHO) data on saturated fat intake of 40 countries shows that the top eight with the *highest* saturated fat consumption, have *lower* rates of heart disease than the eight with the lowest saturated-fat consumption.[3]

Indeed, the American diet itself was rich in saturated animal fats and cholesterol before 1930. Myocardial infarctions (MI)[4] were almost unheard of in the US. In the twenties, there was no name for MI; medical recognition did not exist. However, that doesn't mean there was nothing going on. There *was,* in the fledgling food businesses.

---

[1] See westonaprice.org/knowyourfats/import_sat_fat.html . Also Resources at the back of this book.

[2] Sadly, the misinformation is now so ingrained in most people that neither science nor Scripture can remove it if they are unwilling to receive even the combined truth.

[3] West B, Low Fat Diet: It's Dead – Bury It!, *Health Alert*, Vol. 23, Nr. 9-8, Sept. 2006. See Resources.

[4] A heart attack that occurs when blood supply is severely reduced to the heart muscle (myocardium) as when a blood clot blocks a coronary artery. The affected muscle is called an infarct, thus the term "myocardial infarction." Coronary thrombosis (coronary occlusion) or other terms refer to an obstruction or blockage. Heart attacks may occur for other reasons as well.

During that decade, lucrative "food" manufacturing became two *industries:* highly processed oils, and other foods (white flour, white sugar, white rice, evaporated canned milk, sugary cold cereals, etc.) Manufactured, purified foods extend supermarket shelf life for enhanced merchant profits, not ours. Someone said, "The longer the life of the product, the shorter the life of the consumer."

Living foods, including fresh oils, do not keep for long periods. Hence living components began to be removed from more and more foods. Biogenesis, the assertion that life creates and sustains life ("life begets life"), was rejected.

Actually, vegetable oil began to appear on some store shelves in 1899. Today's refining of cooking/salad oils includes solvent extraction, heating, degumming, bleaching, and deodorizing. During refining, oils are mixed with "an extremely corrosive base," known as "Drano," or another mixture of NaOH and sodium carbonate.[1] Deodorization, a common industrial process for vegetable oils, introduces small amounts of toxic TFA into non-hydrogenated oils.[2]

One would think the original product was replete with unhealthy sediment; whereas the stripped "impurities," as they are referred to in the industry, are the *nutrients* that provide color, odor, and taste (including natural antioxidants vitamins A and E, and vitamin F [essential fatty acids], and other nutrients).[3] With the turn of the twentieth century, except for virgin olive oils, the oils sold at the grocers, were increasingly refined and pure.[4] "Pure" here is related to long shelf life.

It is both tragic and ironic that the removal of nutrients should be equated with "purity." Tragic because if those

---

[1] Erasmus U, *Fats That Heal, Fats That Kill*, Alive Books, 1995:96
[2] Personal email from Dr. Mozaffarian
[3] Sometimes synthetic antioxidants are added to processed oils.
[4] Erasmus, *Ibid.* p. 98 Unprocessed oils should be refrigerated in dark bottles. They will not be thin, clear, and bland, but smell and taste like the seed. Except for virgin olive oils, all the oils at grocers are refined. After experller pressing and solvent extraction, which may allow reaction with light and air to product rancidity, some of the oil may be mixed and marketed as "unrefined." I once purchased and returned rancid oil at a HFS. I haven't used seed oils since.

nutrients were present, they would contribute to the health of the consumer. Ironic, because establishing the desired "purity" really results in producing poor quality food.[1]

Shortening (chemically hardened oil), was first made in 1911. Cheap, devitalized margarine began appearing on America's dinner tables during World War II, as I recall. At first, this white trans fat product came with a perle of orange coloring we kids enjoyed popping and squishing in a plastic bag until this counterfeit looked like butter. Little did my parents know that it and other highly processed foods could lead to the MI that ultimately killed my grandfather. As a first grader, I sat with him during one of his terrifying heart attacks. I shall never forget it...

Erasmus reminds us:

> Business interests are extremely powerful, and affect us all. When the conduct of business is not based on a clear commitment to the common good, it can become dangerous and destructive. The fats and oils business is no exception."[2]

Saturated Fat: Healthy For 6,000 Years

According to hospital records there were no MI deaths recorded from 1868 to 1920.[3] By the late twenties and with the advent of industrial cooking oils, hydrogenated products, and other factory foods, that began to change. By the thirties there were 3,000 deaths per year attributed to coronary thrombosis, now called myocardial infarction (MI), referring to death of part of the heart muscle from lack of oxygen balance from a clot blocking a coronary artery.

In the late twenties when this condition began to surface, the medical treatment was the well-remembered oxygen tent. By 1945,

---

[1] Hawkin P, Rohe F, The History of Vegetable Oil, *Mother Earth News,* Iss. 12, Nov. 1971; 26-27

[2] Erasmus, *Ibid.,* p. 90

[3] Martin W, The Prudent Heart Diet & Cholesterol Lowering Drugs; Why They Don't Prevent Heart Disease – Orthodox Med & Heart Disease; *Townsend Ltrs For Doctors & Patients* Aug-Sep 2002

MI death events had jumped to exponential levels; medical doctors began to treat these patients with low doses of warfarin, the recently discovered blood thinner used to control the rat population by internal bleeding. Vitamin K is essential to clotting and warfarin prevents that action.

By 1950, coronary heart disease was the #1 cause of death in America. Warfarin was failing to prevent second heart attacks.

Not until 1955 was cholesterol associated with heart attacks. Perhaps it was because of a shocking event that year we will discuss next, that dietary cholesterol from saturated fat, was pronounced the cause of MI, lack of evidence notwithstanding. Cardiovascular disease (CVD) related deaths had reached pandemic proportions of approximately half million annually. I recall news reports that even autopsies of American soldiers killed in the Korean War (1950-1953), revealed serious coronary artery plaque in those as young as 18 years old. Saturated fat was blamed.

A Wake-Up Call

President Dwight D. Eisenhower's heart attack in 1955 was a shock to the nation. His Vice-President, Richard Nixon, wisely insisted one of the nation's best cardiologists, Paul Dudley White, MD, be called in from Boston to treat the President. With that special care, Eisenhower recovered from the acute myocardial infarction (MI) and survived six more heart attacks. The good doctor had done all humanly possible, considering the damage and the diet.

The Lipid Hypothesis

The next year, 1956, with this troubling event fresh on the American public's collective mind, the American Heart Association's (AHA) fund raiser was carried live on all the major TV networks all day Sunday. As the parade of authoritative medical and other doctors spoke one by one, the telecast confirmed the nation's worst fear: CVD was the #1 killer disease. No one disagreed with that fact. It wasn't just the President's threatening condition, everyone had a family member or knew someone who suffered heart disease. By the time the formidable lineup were finished informing the country, there was near terror. Who could escape this plague and how?

Not to worry, the cause had been determined. It was carefully explained to children and adults alike that the lipid hypothesis had at last identified the cause for all the viewing world that very day.

An hypothesis implies insufficient evidence for more than a tentative explanation; it derives from a Greek word meaning "to suppose." Yet the impressive medical panel matter-of-factly presented an hypothesis as Gospel truth: saturated fat raises blood cholesterol, causing arterial fatty plaque, leading to heart attacks. It was that simple. End of story.

One difficulty with the hypothesis was and is that though dietary saturated fat continues to decrease, America's #1 cause of death by disease has remained thus for as long as most of its citizens can remember, the numbers being astronomically high and continuing to climb every year since early 1930.

Where were the proof studies demonstrating saturated fat raises everyone's cholesterol (it has never raised ours), that "raised cholesterol" is unhealthy, that it causes arterial fatty plaque; or that this leads to heart attacks? Again, the evidence was lacking.

It was as though the cadiologists had "medical amnesia." Had they forgotten that this new heart disease was discovered in 1925; and for 6,000 years prior to that the diet of the population was replete with saturated fats, including lard, butter, whole milk, meats, and fowl? At the same time they seem to be completely unaware that prior to the seed oil and refined food industries' existence, coronary thrombosis was unknown. How then could they diagnose saturated fats as *bad* and the polyunsaturates as *good?*

They chose to believe that blood clots in the coronary arteries were unrelated to heart attacks. No, it was bad cholesterol from the saturated fat clogging the arteries, thus the name of the disease was changed from coronary thrombosis to myocardial infarction.

Not to worry. The nation was assured that day that a new and delicious cholesterol-lowering diet would successfully remove the problem. Only one doctor there recalled that in the previous 30 years as more and more vegetable oils and hydrogenated fats had been replacing saturated fats on grocers' shelves, that heart disease had not decreased. To the contrary, the numbers were record high and climbing every year.

Is The "Prudent Diet" Really?

Now, to return to the interesting AHA televised event. Having explained the lipid hypothesis, the so-called Prudent Diet (PD) was then very enthusiastically recommended to the nation by the distinguished and trusted panel, including doctors Irving Page, Jeremiah Stamler of the AHA, and researcher Ancel Keys.

Refined vegetable oil, industrially-made margarine and shortening – were to replace natural fats, the all-knowing doctors instructed the trusting populace. Skinless chicken and fish were the recommended flesh foods; red meat was to be entirely avoided. Sugary, cold cereal processed with high temperatures, eaten with low-fat milk, and other high carb, processed foods, became breakfast. Eggs were out.

The panel, which should have thoroughly investigated the long-term effects of these altered dietary recommendations, pronounced them "health foods" to replace natural cooking fats[1], beef, butter, bacon,[2] and eggs.

With projected profits likely to exceed all records since the food industry's establishment, it was no doubt in ecstasy. However, one notable member of the panel was anything but pleased!

To promote further trust, the glowing MC then turned to Dr. White, the President's cardiologist, and asked the good doctor to tell of the great success medical doctors were experiencing with solving heart disease issues. Obviously the MC had not spoken with Dr. White before the show.

---

[1] We do not use lard for other reasons. We cook with EV olive oil and unrefined coconut butter.
[2] We are not endorsing pork.

The highly proclaimed cardiologist said that antibiotics had greatly reduced syphilis (STD) related heart attacks, but other than that there had been a major increase in MI deaths.

The medical specialist then showed the TV camera a small worn book entitled "A Treatise on Sudden Death" written by two medical doctors at Oxford University in 1860. The book told of two rare deaths, the etiology of which were a complete mystery then. We would recognize them today, nearly a century later, as MI, he said. Dr. White then asked the question of the century: "What did people eat back then - when death from myocardial infarction almost never happened - but butter, lard, and high cholesterol food?"

Concerning the new "miracle diet," Dr. White argued that MIs were non-existent in 1900 when egg consumption was three times what it was then (1956)! With 35 years of close observation and experience with patients' coronary health, when pressured to endorse the PD, he would tolerate no more of the nonsense. Boldly rising to the occasion, he sprang to his feet, and exclaimed:

> See here! I began my practice as a cardiologist in 1921 and never saw a myocardial infarction patient until 1928. Back in the MI-free days…the fats were [saturates] butter, whole milk, and lard; and I think we would all benefit from the kind of diet we had when no one ever heard of corn oil!

Asked Phil Handler, former president of the National Academy of Sciences:

> What right has the federal government to propose that the American people conduct a vast nutritional experiment with themselves as subjects, on the strength of so very little evidence that it will do them any good?

Did Handler suspect the profound harm to be wrought upon the country? "All reformers would do well to be conscious of the law of unintended consequences," said Alan Stone, staff director for Senator George McGovern's committee on low-fat hearings.

The consequences with this "vast nutritional experiment" were inconceivable and profoundly immeasurable.

If only the world had heeded those words of wisdom...Indeed, statistics, logic, decades of experience, and a few but strong studies were on the good doctor's side. Timing was not. A recent Russian study seemed to support the lipid hypothesis. It found that rabbits fed saturated fat in their vegetarian ration, developed arterial plaque. Never mind that these vegetarian animals naturally consume only plants, and humans are naturally omnivorous; meaning that fats are not naturally a part of rabbits' diets, whereas they are essential for humans.

More appropriate would have been the publishing of the 1956 Harvard study done with dogs; which like humans, consume saturates. After 3.5-4 years of blood cholesterol maintained at 495-570 mg.%, very careful "...autopsy failed to reveal any abnormalities in the cardiovascular system or liver."[1]

A medical doctor known to us, speaks of having had one 50 minute nutrition class in medical school. Trained chiefly in the use of pharmaceuticals, surgery, radiation, and chemotherapy, most medics are happy to leave nutrition to the nutritionists. However, the medical standard of care had not solved the gargantuan problem. Researcher Ancel Keys was very convincing with his selective international study and other flawed ones that appeared to point to the Prudent Diet as the ideal solution.

For years before Dr. White's courageous stand that night, nutrition pioneers had argued in vain with the government against devitalized foods. Even the first director of the FDA did not allow interstate sales of such foods.

As experienced and knowledgeable as was Dr. White regarding heart disease and the consequences of altered foods, his old fashioned, evidence-based opinion regarding the traditional diet, was rejected. Chiefly the timing of Key's study and the Russian one (later invalidated), with their seemingly scientific and sound conclusions, were sufficient to persuade the medical community of the validity of the lipid hypothesis.

---

[1] Shull KH, Mann GV, Response of Dogs to Long-Term Cholesterol Feeding, *Am J Physiol* 188: 81-85, 1956;

In 1620, at the same time as the Plymouth Colony was being established by the Pilgrims, British statesman, philosopher and attorney Francis Bacon described the case succinctly as few have:

> The human understanding when it has once adopted an opinion (either as being the received opinion or as being agreeable to itself) draws all things else to support and agree with it. And though there be a greater number and weight of instances to be found on the other side, yet these it either neglects and despises, or else by some distinction sets aside and rejects, in order that by this great and pernicious predetermination the authority of its former conclusions may remain inviolate.[1]

Human nature has not changed since Adam and certainly not since Bacon observed this principle. Once the mind is made up about a matter, many people see only what supports what they believe, or they interpret it thus.

As experienced and knowledgeable as was Dr. White regarding heart disease, and the consequences of altered foods, his old fashioned and evidence-based opinion regarding the proven traditional diet, was rejected. "…[F]atally flawed by selection bias and confounding variables, the 'conclusions,' which were actually inferences, were widely accepted…Healthcare workers and policy makers were generally unaware of the concept of evidence-based medicine, let alone the rigor of Level 1 evidence; that is, prospective, randomized human studies," wrote Gil Wilshire, MD, FACOG.[2]

It was supposed to be oh so simple: stop consuming saturated fats; start eating polyunsaturates (vegetable oils), and more carbs. By the time TVs were turned off that day, surely ill-advised medics were as excited as race horses at the gate, chomping at the bit to prescribe the newly named diet for their atherosclerotic and MI

---

[1] *Novum Organum*,
[2] *Weight of the Evidence*,
weightoftheevidence.blogspot.com/2006_06_01_archive

patients who had suffered at least one heart attack.[1] To launch the Prudent Diet, supportive organizational literature parroted the lipid hypothesis and the AHA panel's misinformation and recommendations. The food industry distributed millions of pieces of propaganda as to how healthy it all was, even margarine and shortening!

Seemingly few of the medical doctors realized that the so-called Prudent Diet was anything *but*. In fact, the diet has been shown to guarantee cardiovascular diseases will be around as long as it is. Fifty years after its "coming-out party," instead of the then 600,000 MI deaths annually, the staggering toll has skyrocketed to nearly one million today.[2]

Please do not misunderstand, I am not anti-medicine. There is need for both natural and allopathic health care. Some very good friends are compassionate Christian and non-Christian medical doctors of sterling character, whom I respect. They are excellent diagnosticians. When I require medical care I consult them. They also respect me, my health choices, skills, 40 years of research, and training. We have successfully worked together for years.

I know medics highly esteme medical science. And yet alarmed and disturbed medical doctor Wilshire further declares: "…the fact [is] that in the past half century NOT ONE SMIDGEN OF LEVEL 1 EVIDENCE HAS BEEN GENERATED TO SUPPORT THESE [PD] RECOMMENDATIONS.[3] I don't know how to say it any louder or clearer."

Incredibly, in 2006 the AHA updated its dietary guidelines for heart health to recommend a further reduction of saturated fat to less than 7% of calories. Doubling of polyunsaturates over saturates did not decrease MI deaths. *Au contraire.* Unless simultaneously reduced trans fats improves the numbers, this higher polyunsaturate:saturate ratio will further increase the death

---

[1] If it seems to you that conventional nutritionists and medical doctors, public health authorities, TV, the Internet, various literature – from professional journals to slick health magazines – still do today, it's not your imagination.

[2] When the profound cost of MIs are considered, few think of the survivors' loss, e.g., the grandchildren's. A friend wrote: "I was thinking…how we were robbed of my godly grandmother at age 65 when she had a…heart attack… How I would love to have known her better."

[3] Emphasis in the original.

toll from CVD if the 75 years of history is any indication.

Beef, Butter & Eggs Versus Big Money

Clearly logic alone would not have allowed the acceptance of the unsound diet considering that heart disease was almost non-existent when saturated fats were the chief fats. Having quickly accepted an hopothesis as scientific fact, and the PD as America's best hope in spite of "so little evidence that the vast nutritional experiment" would succeed, those in the health care community *then* set out to clinically prove its effectiveness.[1] Doesn't that seem backwards and that the proof should have come first?

Most importantly, almost overnight the nation's cardiologists came to complete faith in the diet. Sheer desperation it appears, prevailed over sound reasoning; requirement for extensive scientific proof flew out the window. The PD locked in CVD as the number one cause of morbidity and mortality in the nation, as wishful thinking won over evidence-based wisdom.

Over a period of decades, the food industry's slick ads and labels had been effectively weaning America from non-hydrogenated, animal-based fats, coconut and palm oils. Industrially-altered products carried claims of health benefits, and were less expensive. Their low costs had priced real foods almost off the grocers' shelves. And after all, the government wouldn't allow them to sell us anything that wasn't healthy, and our health care community wouldn't advise us to eat it otherwise, right? Surely they meant well even as today when the same is recommended.

Unreasonable bias against red meat and animal fats quickly became a stronghold in the nation that if anything, is increasing today. That saturated fats were causing heart attacks and deaths by the millions over the decades was doubted by fewer and fewer as time went on and the reinforcing of the idea permeated not just the health care community but everywhere from the pulpit to the porch.

---

[1] Scientifically, experimentation or continued observation support or refute most hypotheses. The lipid hypothesis and PD were refuted long ago.

Increased replacement of so many of God's wholesome foods with man's nutrient-deficient ones, has not only significantly enhanced profits for patented foods, it has also resulted in unintentional corresponding benefits for burgeoning health and related industries, as CVD and certain other patients have multiplied exponentially.[1] (From very few CVD deaths in 1925, the US figure catapulted to more than half million MI-related funerals in 1960 to almost double that in 2006. The countless costs and losses associated with MI deaths, and that long term illness, are impossible to calculate or comprehend.)

The permitted foods of the PD were not new; remember, "factory foods" had been around since before the twenties. What was different was that people were now to stop eating all animal-based foods (especially beef, butter, and eggs) except skim milk for cold cereal, and to eat instead, many more fabricated foods containing highly processed vegetable oils, including cooking and salad oils, shortening, margarine, white flour and sugar.

It was so easy and exciting for grocery-shopping housewives to find advertised beautifully packaged new products which boldly displayed labels clearly stating "**NO CHOLESTEROL!**" and "**HEART HEALTHY**," (no saturated fat), even as now. (Today's oils are in cheaper plastic bottles rather than glass which has no chemicals.)

It seems the dynamic of such an eating plan is, "If what you're eating is making you ill, then eat more of it to get well." It would be laughable but for the potential of becoming the greatest destroyer of life and productivity of all time.

This is not to say that CVD is caused by diet alone. There surely are other contributing factors. However, I have observed that exercise, reduced stress, and other lifestyle improvements cannot overcome the PD with its heavy reliance on manufactured foods, especially polyunsaturates and other "faux-foods."

There is an exception I have also noted: a good genome can keep one alive to amazing old age.[2] Yet even in those cases, individuals (and their parents), ate mostly wholesome, fresh diets, if only in childhood.

---

[1] Erasmus, *Ibid,*, p. 99. Consider also other diet-related diseases.
[2] A genome is the total genetic information stored in 23 pairs of chromosomes

PART II

Study The Studies

We will be considering the results of a number of remarkable studies in this chapter and others. Not all studies "are created equal." It is important to know and understand details of how the studies are carried out. They may have been flawed or limited in their value. Did they study large populations historically (descriptive, less definitive), or groups for a period of time (cohort)? Are they case controlled (memory reliance); or randomized trials (considered by many to be the "gold standard") where separate groups are selected randomly, and fed certain foods or not for a period of time; after which the results are compared.

Check Them Out!

The newspapers reports of the Joliffe study were not wrong; neither did they nearly tell the whole truth, so that they were actually very misleading. It was necessary to read the actual study to get the alarming truth. Reading only the study extract may not tell you what vital facts. Here is an example of omission of information from the study extracts that is pertinent to an accurate conclusion:

Some studies showing saturated fat causes atherosclerosis were performed using products full of chemicals and additives that were responsible for the results. All saturated fat is not the same. So-called "junk meats" such as processed, cured, and ready-to-use, lunch meats; wieners, sausages, and bacon, instead of fresh meats, were used. Down south in Argentina where they grow a tremendous amount of grass-fed beef, a recent study confirmed there is a vast difference between clean, red meat (the Creator provided), and man-made meat products with as much as 37% ground fat mixed with nitrosamines and other preservatives and additives.

"They Did Not Listen…They're Not Listening Still…"

Norman Joliffe, MD, director of New York City's Nutrition Bureau and founder of the Anticoronary Club, directed the first of a long line of studies with the PD. His study was expected to prove the diet would rid the US of its death-dealing plague of MI's.

Half of Dr. Joliffe's study's participants were men ranging in age from 40-59 years old who were members of the Anticoronary Club. They consumed the PD's corn oil, shortening, margarine, skinless chicken, and sugary cereal. The other half of his subjects enjoyed red meat, butter, lard, bacon, and eggs with great gusto. Both the PD consumers and the red meat eaters included plenty of carbohydrates in their diets, including refined ones.

Obese and confined to a wheelchair, Dr. Jolliffe was a "vascular wreck." Blind in one eye, he suffered a diabetic ulcer on one foot. He had complete confidence the PD would not only prevent further complications, including heart disease, but would also cure his his tragic condition. Yet he died of "diabetic complications" (vascular thrombosis – blood clots) before the four year study ended. Had one of the clots reached his heart, he might have died of a MI.

The Joliffe study was "hailed as a great success" for the PD because the serum cholesterol of those participants was reduced from 225 mg.% to 200 mg.% during the six years of the study.[1] This newspaper headline ran for about a week, interpreted to mean that the Prudent Diet would prevent heart attacks since it was claimed "high cholesterol" was the cause of them. There was jubilation!

What the public was not told was that the study also showed that besides the director of the study, eight other participants who consumed the PD suffered fatal heart attacks, while *none* of the subjects died who ate saturated fat. Dr. Joliffe could well have said, "We're going to lower your cholesterol if it kills you!"

---

[1] *Jnl. of the Amer Med Assn*; Nov. 7, 1966:129-134

Remember, half of heart patients don't have "high" cholesterol. Regardless, was the goal to lower cholesterol or to avoid a MI? Would you rather have been in the lower cholesterol group or the group with no deaths?

Actually, the nutritionally inadequate PD is full of hidden spoilers that may lead to health erosion over time. As you will see in the review of the following reports, the first sign of the diet's invisible work is sometimes a drop-dead heart attack, or a MI that leaves one facing long term illness. I have personally known two medical doctors and knew of two others who were believed to be in perfect health, who considered that diet to be very healthy, yet they all died suddenly of MI's.

The National Heart Study That Failed Before Launching

Next, Irvine H. Page, MD, member of the distinguished American Heart Association TV panel who had survived a heart attack, proposed the National Heart Study of a million men across the nation. He too was confident it would be an "utter success" for him personally, and it would settle the heart disease issue for most of the nation for all time.

Wayne Martin, cancer researcher, told of his meeting with Dr. Page at the time this trial was in the planning stage. "He was utterly confident that the Prudent Diet was going to keep him from having another heart attack. He was also expressing his sorrow for the several thousands of…controls who were expected to die of heart attacks. He said that he expected…very few such deaths among the subjects on the Prudent Diet."[1]

"Such a distinguished post-coronary scientific savant as Dr. Page, likes to quip that he still follows a low fat, low cholesterol diet because he has no intention of being the smartest man in the cemetary. The evidence indicates he will not be that," responded Professor George Mann.[2]

The study was to be directed by the AHA and US government funding of millions of dollars. Taxpayers' dollars were used setting

---

[1] Martin W, The Prudent Heart Diet and Cholesterol Lowering Drugs; why they don't prevent heat disease, *Townsend Ltrs For Doctors & Pts,* Aug-Sep 2002,
[2] Groves B, Second Opinion, secondopinions.co.uk/ as viewed 3/17/07

up food warehouses in seven cities where the men would be able to get the non-fresh PD foods free for this monmouth study, including donuts saturated with polyunsatures and made with refined flour and sugar.

The Modern Family Cookbook, my first cookbook, purchased in 1953, further reflects the incredibly successful indoctrination of the food industry:

> It is no longer necessary to force whole wheat bread and whole wheat flour on people who prefer white. During Word War II most white flour was enriched by the addition of certain vitamins and iron, making it more nearly equal in food value to the whole wheat flour...It is therefore less essential today that people learn to like whole wheat bread, because they can get the vitamins and much of the mineral content from white breads made with enriched flour.[1]

Then listing the comparatively few vitamin isolates plus iron "added back" to the "enriched flour," it states, "All these elements are present in the germ and other parts of the wheat kernel which are discarded in the refining process." If a thousand dollars were stolen from you and the thief returned three dollars, would you consider yourself to be "enriched"?

Before the huge National Heart Study was to be carried out, a pretrial with 2,000 men was run for three years. It too ended in "utter failure" for the PD.

The men consuming saturated fat were also eating processed foods that did not contain vegetable oils and hydrogenated fats but were high in simple, refined carbs. The pretrial results ended with no fewer heart attacks with the PD.[2] Judging from other studies, but for the refined carbs, there would very likely have been far fewer deaths in the saturate fat-eating group. Much later, the Mozaffarian study revealed the significance of this. Later we will discuss that very important study.

---

[1] Givens M, *The Modern Family Cookbook, J. G.* Ferguson & Assoc., Chicago, 1953:88-89

[2] *The Lancet,* 1968:ii:693

Dr. Page, who had been very confident he would never have another heart attack while consuming the PD, nevertheless died of this while consuming that diet, as Professor Mann had predicted.

The National Heart Study, introduced with great fanfare, was quietly cancelled "for reasons of cost." No more was said about it. However, in the UK another study at that time produced the same results as the Page pre-trial. Once again, the PD produced no improvement in heart attacks.[1] And once again the authoritative health community was blind to the obvious truth. It has continued to recommend the diet as a "heart healthy" one.

If At First You Don't Succeed…

After the National Heart Study was cancelled, five population studies were conducted with cities that previously had consumed almost entirely saturated fat as the only fat, with low incidence of heart disease. Unimpeachable evidence showed that after beginning the PD, within 15 years or less there were 65% more heart attacks. Incredibly, these unexpected facts were filed away and the trusting public never told.

An interesting one of those studies, the Boston Irish Brothers Study in 1965, included pairs of brothers, half of them living in the US, the other half in Ireland. The brothers in Ireland continued to consume a diet with large amounts of saturated fat from animal-source foods. Fred Stare, MD, cardiologist at Harvard University School of Public Health, found that the average adult in Ireland ate more than a pound of butter a week and "almost none of the GOOD polyunsaturated vegetable oil or margarines in diet."[2]

Again it was expected that the brothers in Boston consuming the PD (as almost the entire nation basically has been doing since 1960), would have far fewer MI deaths. Just the opposite occurred! This study too was ignored by the media, medics, and government alike. Instead, the Irish were said to walk more than their American brothers, and cardiologists attributed the difference to that.[3]

---

[1] *Lancet,* 1968:ii:693-6
[2] Martin W, *Townsend Ltrs For Drs & Pts.,* Aug-Sep 2002
[3] Second Opinion, UK; http://www.second-opinions.co.uk/martin_chd.html

A study reported in the *American Journal of Clinical Nutrition* was performed comparing North India, the "world's biggest butter eaters," with South India which followed the PD "more closely than anyone in the USA." The latter experienced 15 times more MI deaths compared to the butter-fat consuming North Indians.[1]

After switching to the cheap vegetable oils and margarine, the mortality rate of men and women of North India rose to equal the South Indian one.[2]

In a recent report of a study of TV "junk food" commercials aimed at children and teens, it was lamented that poultry and seafood were not mentioned in the commercials. Yet obviously absent from the study-recommended foods for a wholesome diet were meat and dairy products.

Though some whole foods are now emphasized, many counterfeit foods of the Prudent Diet still come directly from the fabricated-food industry to replace animal-source ones.[3] By recommending vegetable oils, margarines, egg substitutes, low-fat milk, skinless chicken, soy and nut "milks," high-carb cold cereals, and other non-whole, processed products, the health care industry, including conventional nutritionists and dieticians, have provided the "food" industry its credibility and enhanced its proftability for over half a century

A growing body of scientific research reveals the fact of increased deaths of strokes and heart attacks "...in direct proportion to the increase in **polyunsaturated** fats in our diet," observed scientist Wayne Martin. In a British study involving several thousand men, half were asked to reduce saturated fat and cholesterol in their diets, to stop smoking and to increase the amounts of unsaturated oils such as margarine and vegetable oils. After one year, those on the so called "good" diet had 100 percent *more* deaths than those on the "bad" diet who smoked![4]

---

[1] Malhotra SL, *Amer Jnl of Clin Nutr*, vol. 20, May 1967, pp. 462-74
[2] Raheja B, Ghee, *Lancet*, Ghee, cholesterol and heart disease; Nov. 14, 1987-114
[3] Only God can create real foods.
[4] Rose, G, et al, *The Lancet*, 1:1983;1062-1065

Amazing "Blue Ribbon" Studies

New evidential scientific studies are also most revealing. One of these reported in the *American Journal of Clinical Nutrition* was a very important multifaceted study directed by Harvard's Dariush Mozaffarian, MD.[1] Dr. Mozaffarian is a cardiologist with training in epidemiology and nutrition. His objective was "to investigate associations between dietary macronutrients and progression of coronary atherosclerosis among post-menopausal women." This Brigham and Women's Hospital's three year study involved 235 American women averaging 66 years of age at the beginning. All the participants had arterial plaque.

Each participant's heart arteries were X-rayed at 10 different locations at the beginning and end of the study. Amazingly, after three years, "…those women who had **regularly eaten the highest amounts of saturated fats had the least amount of additional plaque build-up in their arteries."**

These were the last people we would expect to improve on such a diet. They were overweight/obese, 19-31% of whom were diabetic, 66% taking sex hormones,[2] overweight/obese, with skewed blood fats, and hypertensive, "consistent with metabolic syndrome." Yet they experienced *diminished* coronary artery disease progression when fat intake was highest in saturates, not lowest; *reducing* a major complication millions of others also suffer.

The study appears to show *exactly the opposite of what we have been told for decades about saturated fats, cholesterol, atherosclerosis, and MI*[3] There were no deaths during the study.

---

[1] Mozaffarian D, Rimm EB, Herrington DM, Dietary fats, carbohydrate, and progression of coronary atherosclerosis in postmenopausal women. *Am J Clin Nutr* 2004;80:1175-1184

[2] "The failure of sex hormones to prevent coronary artery disease has been a great disappointment," according to an AJCN editorial by Knopp amd Retzaff entitled "Saturated fat prevents coronary artery disease? An American paradox," Amer Jnl of Clncl Nutr; Vol. 80, No. 5, 1102-1103, Nov. 2004.

[3] Kinsell LW, Michaels GD, Cochrane GC, Partridge JW, Jahn JP, Balch HE. Effect of vegetable fat on hypercholesterolemia and hyperphospholipidemia: observations on diabetic and nondiabetic subjects given diets high in vegetable fat and protein. Diabetes 1954;3:113-9

What did medical science do with such invaluable knowledge you might ask. It is disappointing this remarkable study is deemed to be a "paradox...found **in women with the metabolic syndrome**..." [1] Next you will learn of a number of studies using male participants only or both men and women.

Following the flawed Russian rabbit study, an often quoted Finnish mental hospital diet of the sixties reported dramatic drops in coronary artery disease (CAD) with vegetable oils. The Mozaffarian *et al* study demonstrated the opposite association; it "found a **higher saturated fat intake** is associated with **less progresson of coronary artery disease**..." according to quantitative angiography - almost exactly the same as the city-wide Framingham heart study. The latter study has been carried on for generations with men and women, where the glaring fact is that "...**[T]he more saturated fat one ate, the more cholesterol one ate..., the *lower* the person's serum cholesterol**..."[2]

Another Finnish study of 1,930 men concluded in 1997: "**There was no association between intakes of saturated [fat,]...dietary cholesterol, and the risk of coronary deaths.**" [3]

Even so, conventionally "It is an article of faith that saturated fat raises LDL cholesterol and accelerates coronary artery disease, whereas unsaturated fatty acids have the opposite effect," according to conventional medical science.[4] In this context a non-religious article of faith is an unshakable, accepted belief *requiring no proof or evidence* [how scientific is this?], and is simply *not to be doubted* [and this?].

Has the passing of half a century of itself transformed ingrained, unsubstantiated non-truth into an "article of faith" comparable with a proven such as the earth is round? Did the fact that medical doctors did not believe in the existence of germs and refused to wash their hands after autopsies before delivering babies, prevent the pathogenic deaths of mothers of new borns?

---

[1] Knopp RH, Retzlaff B, *Op. cit.* .
[2] Castelli, WP, *Archives of Intrnl Med,* 1992:152:1371-2
[3] Pietinen P, Ascherio A, *et al,* Intake of fatty acids and risk of coronary heart disease in a cohort of Finnish Men; The Alpha-Tocopherol, Beta Carotene Cancer Prevention Study; Amer Jnl Epidemiol 1997 May 15;145(10):876-87
[4] Knopp and Retzlaff, *Op Cit.*

Yet the conventional mindset presumes saturated leads to "high" cholesterol (whatever that may be at the moment), causes heart disease; and that polyunsaturated fats have the opposite effect in the general population.

Saturated fat has not raised our extended blended family's cholesterol, or that of patients and clients I have taught the Creator's fresh, whole-foods diet for almost as long as the PD has been put forth. I have also witnessed decreased cholesterol levels when the PD or vegan diet is changed to avoid processed foods and include saturated fats from animal-source foods, coconut oil and fresh coconut. In my opinion the above noted Mozaffarian *et al* study supports this observation.

Other Harvard studies have shown "…**there is only a weak relationship between the amount of cholesterol a person consumes and their blood cholesterol levels**, or **risk for heart disease**." [1] Other studies confirm those facts, as did the Hayes study mentioned below. Actually, high blood cholesterol levels protected chronic heart failure patients in a UK study, "…leading to dramatic reductions in death rates."

Second, since "safe levels" are continually being lowered, how do we know that anyone knows what truly is safe? We *do* know what is presently considered to be low cholesterol is *un*safe.[2]

Third, there is a great deal of evidence to show saturated fat does not cause heart disease in the general population as we have shown in this book and other referenced works.

Mary Enig, PhD, who literally wrote the book on fatty acids,[3] and who is a highly respected expert on the subject, has for years testified:

> The idea that saturated fats cause heart disease is completely wrong, but the statement has been "published" so many times over the last three or more decades that it is very difficult to convince people otherwise unless they

---

[1] hsph.harvard.edu/nutritionsource/fats.html as viewed Mar. 5, 2007
[2] My research revealed countless studies pointing to various cancers with this group.
[3] *Know Your Fats.* See Resources.

are willing to take the time to read and learn what...produced the anti-saturated fat agenda. [1]

In another Harvard Medical School study published in the *Journal of the American Medical Association,* Mathew Gillman, MD, *et al*, showed that "a diet high in polyunsaturated fats is associated with increased risk of thrombotic stroke as compared to a diet high in saturated fat."[2]

We do not buy low-fat products, including dairy products.[3] Though most Americans believe this saturated fat has been associated with CVD, whole milk did not increase the risk in a study of first acute MI's reported in the *British Medical Journal* in 2004.[4]

"The women [in the Mozaffarian study] who ate more saturated fat also had **a healthier balance of good and bad cholesterols, as well as more desirable blood concentrations of various kinds of fats.**" Dr. White – may he rest in peace - would have shouted, "Of course!" Perhaps this is in part due to a like increase in HDL.

Harvard studies have shown "...there is only a weak relationship between the amount of cholesterol a person consumes and their blood cholesterol levels, **or risk for heart disease**."[5] Other studies confirm that fact, as did the Hayes study.

Why have we not heard of these studies over and over as we did the flawed rabbit and other studies demeaning saturated fat for more than 60 years? Why were such studies not performed well *before* the PD was presented to the nation as *the* solution for its horrendous problem with cardiovascular disease? Why does the AHA still insist that "saturated fat is the main dietary cause of high blood cholesterol"?

And why have the media and press not responded aggressively as they "picked up the ball" and have been running with it since

---

[1] Enig, M, Diet, Serum Cholesterol and Coronary Heart Disease; Mann G, editorial, Coronary Heart Disease. 1993
[2] Gillman M, et al, *Jnl. Amer Med Assn,* Dec. 24, 1987:2145-50
[3] We purchase almost no industrially manufactured foods.
[4] Warensjo E, *et al, British Jnl of Nutr* 91(4):635-642, April 2004.
[5] hsph.harvard.edu/nutritionsource/fats.html as viewed Mar. 5, 2007

1956 toward the wrong goal? Their silence is deafening when it comes to these extremely important and most credible studies. Can you think of reasons for this?

Even the USDA's food pyramid, heavy on carbs, remains unchanged in the face of these shocking facts. One of its websites, *Choose A Diet Low In Fat, Saturated Fat, And Cholesterol*, advises eating carbs *"because they are low in fats."* It even recommends choosing vegetable oils and soft margarine for these![1] We pay tax dollars for this "head in the sand" blindness.

Remember the preliminary study published in the Mayo Proceedings regarding insulin-driven hypertension as also reported by endocrinologist James H. Hayes, MD at the 2006 annual conference of clinical endocrinologists? Those participants were allowed "free range" of meat and saturated fats, while no starches were permitted.[2]

Many believe fat, especially saturated fat, causes obesity. For starters, the participants in this study consumed half pound of bacon plus a half dozen eggs **per day** for breakfast. Yet even with a very high saturated fat intake (double the usual recommendation), rapid **weight loss** occurred without the high carbs.

The "patients achieved significant improvements in hypertension and a number of CVD risk factors...," including **reductions in blood lipid levels** and significant increases in HDL and LDL particle sizes. While the lack of starchy foods is a large factor, clearly the results of the study fly in the face of the lipid hypothesis and PD which insist that saturated fat increases blood cholesterol.[3] "Most of what you think you know . . . just isn't so. Consider the facts, check the references, and dare to think" for yourself," said Darlene Sherrell.

PD's High Risk High Carbs

For more than five decades, not only has the PD *not* cured the **#1** killer, it is associated with a circle of degenerative diseases that

---

[1] http://www.nal.usda.gov/fnic/dga/dga95/grains.html
[2] Breads, cereals, rices, pasta, potatoes, et al.
[3] CAUTION: This diet should not be undertaken except under a physician's care.

is being perilously enlarged over the years. As long as our food touts "LOW FAT," "NO CHOLESTEROL" we don't care what else might be in it.

Though the World Health Organization (WHO) has recommended that industrialized countries consume low-glycemic index foods in order to prevent coronary heart disease, diabetes and obesity, sugar remains a major part of the PD, beginning with cereal and high carb breakfasts.

Not only do cancers thrive on sugar, carbohydrates such as corn and grain, when fed to cattle, create very thick cover fat and marbling in the muscles. Could a diet high in carbs be associated with an accumulation of atheroma and plaque in human arteries? The Mozaffarian complex study referenced herein, revealed another dietary imbalance may be significant.

Very importantly, Dr. Mozaffarian and Harvard had the wisdom and courage to consider also the carbohydrate intake of the participants in relation to the plaque progression, making the study doubly valuable with the second *critical* piece of the puzzle.

"The women with the **highest amounts of carbs** in their diet for the three year study, **had the most plaque build-up.**" Imagine the effects of a lifetime of high carbs.

In that study, it was *not* saturated fats, but high carbs, and especially refined carbs, that are associated with "the number one killer of Americans" year after year, millions upon millions.[1] (Vegetable oils were not a part of this study though Dr. Mozaffarian has taken a stand against trans fats.)

Contrary to the Russian rabbit study and some others,[2] the conclusion of this cited study, was that "...***greater saturated fat intake*** **is associated with** *less* **progression of coronary atherosclerosis, whereas** *carbohydrate intake* **is associated with a** *greater* **progression.**"

If increased saturated fat slows this progression and high amounts of carbs increases it, might it be beneficial if we consume lesser amounts of carbs, and enjoy "greater saturated fat intake" in animal-based foods beginning in childhood?

---

[1] More on this in *Eatin' After Eden – God's Whole Menu*
[2] Enig & Fallon, "The Oiling of America," westonaprice.org/knowyourfats/oiling.

Vegetable Oils: One Way They Increase Cholesterol

Increased consumption of polyunsaturated acids (vegetable oils) since World War II, has produced changes in hormones in the general population, according to Ray Peat, Ph.D., Professor Emeritus of Endocrinology at the University of Oregon.

> Their best understood effect is their interference with the function of the thyroid gland. Unsaturated oils block thyroid hormone secretion, its movement in the circulatory system, and the response of tissues to the hormone...The thyroid hormone is required for using and eliminating cholesterol, so cholesterol is likely to be raised by anything which blocks the thyroid function [including soy and raw cruciferous vegetables].[1]

Rancid Oils

Except for extra virgin olive oil, there is a tremendous difference in fresh, nutrient-rich seed oil the Creator put there and what we find in plastic bottles lining supermarket shelves today. When the processing is complete, the various odors and tastes of the original oils are gone (along with the nutrients) so that we don't smell the rancidity. Destructive free radicals are odorless in these very unstable polyunsaturates both in the unopened bottle and after bringing them home. Even before cooking, at room temperature, and exposing to air oxygen when removing the lid of the bottle, oxidation accelerates. Cooking with vegetable oils greatly exacervates the oxidation rate and free radical formation.

Rancid oils from seeds, soy beans, summer rolled oats, brown rice, and processed foods with vegetable oils, are chief sources of free radicals, and may lead to the serious diseases associated with these. We avoid these completely and commercial and restaurant salad dressings.

---

[1] Peat R, Unsaturated Vegetable Oils Are Toxic, *Raymond Peat Newsletter*, 1996.

On the other hand, olive oil, with its high monosaturates, may be used to cook with at low temperatures though I chiefly use it for salads. Unrefined coconut butter/oil is high in stable saturates[1] and may be ued for medium and high heat below 350^0, though I usually cook at low temperature, and high heat never.

Vegetable Oil Consumption & Wrinkles

The first thing one notices upon approaching Lennie is her unusually wrinkled face. Women who consume mostly vegetable oils often have far more wrinkles than those who eat traditional animal fats, according to some plastic surgeons.[2]

Lennie, who has carefully avoided saturated fat for many years, ultimately came very near death from hypercoagulation and hypertension. Her blood was extremely thick (not uncommon with vegans and those consuming trans fats), and she developed high blood pressure. Animal-source cod liver oil has been shown to support the body's production of slippery platelets. It contains EPA, DHA, and vitamins A and D, all of which are required for a healthy cardiovascular system. Caviar (fish eggs/roe) is also rich in vital Omega 3.[3]

By the way, smoking increases wrinkles by 200-300 percent. Worse, as many as 30 percent of all CVD deaths in the US each year are attributable to cigarette smoking – all preventable. [4]

If Saturated Fat Is The Culprit...

Eve wasn't the only one deceived about what to eat. Ask anyone you know what *they* know about saturated fat and they will usually say something like, "It comes from beef and dairy products

---

[1] Coconut oils med. chain fatty acids are helpful, not harmful to the body.
[2] Enig & Fallon, The Oiling of America, WAPF, 1999
[3] According to a study reported in *Int Jnl of Cancer*, Mar. 1, 2002, women who ate the most omega 3 foods had 1/3 the breast ca. risk of those who ate the least. A 1999 NZ study *et al* showed a 40% lower incidence of prostate ca. with EPA.
[4] marthajefferson.org/modules/cardiac/smoke.htm is an excellent website for smoking stats.

and eggs. They have cholesterol that causes heart disease. We shouldn't eat those foods, maybe only low fat dairy foods."

They are certain there is scientific proof of these "facts." Actually, most of the "scientific evidence" evolves from the unscientific lipid hypothesis, and flawed studies setting out to validate that theory. While many no longer understand the need to prove anything; we all should just accept what they have.

Besides all the studies, we have testimonies, including those of medics, who lived during the period of 1875 to 1960. Then there's Dr. White's national TV declaration in 1956, plus statistics that the world had no MI until well into the last century.

Let's look at it another way: if saturated fat is the culprit, the dietary intake from beef, and butter (which *fell* 85%), should have soared along with the hundreds of thousands of obituaries. Right? Instead, dietary cholesterol intake increased only a fraction during the first half of last century, while refined vegetable oil intake including margarine, shortening, and salad oil, increased approximately 300%, about the same percentage of increase in MI deaths for the period. Those numbers are just the opposite of what we should expect to find if what we have been led to believe is true!

PART III

Trans Fatty Acids – Included In God's Good Foods?

*Wherefore do ye spend money for that which is not bread [food]? And your labor for that which satisfies not? Hearken diligently unto me, and eat ye that which is **good**, and let your soul delight itself in fatness...*[1]
*...[He] satisfies thy mouth with **good** things, so that thy youth is renewed like the eagles...*[2]

The Creator's "good things" renew us. Yet when those whole foods are radically altered by man they can and do have the opposite effect since our bodies are not designed for that metabolism.

Many people don't care for fish, or they are steering away from it now due to the mercury scare.[3] With the PD, that leaves tasteless, skinless chicken; fruits, vegetables, and countless industrially-manufactured foods for lunch and dinner. Most Americans eat few fruits, usually only a banana now and then, and no vegetables except toxic French fries which probably have no nutrients. How many times a week can one enjoy chicken before eating mostly "factory-foods"? And eating them they are!

Most of these foods include processed vegetable oils or partially hydrogenated oils, extreme alterations of vegetable oils containing trans fatty acid (TFA or trans fat), chiefly from soy. (The unhydrogenated vegetable oils also contain a small amount of more toxic TFA as previously noted.)

Artificially hardened oils have no nutrients and provide no benefit to our health. In fact, there is nothing good about this

---

[1] Isa. 55:2
[2] Psa. 103:5
[3] Yet those who don't eat fish will often devour "junk food."

"faux-fat;" but much that is not. Along with some nutritious foods, the PD includes worse than nutrient-deficient foods laden with hidden toxins, e.g. TFA, the "Trojan Horse of the food industry."

The All-Pervasive Counterfeit

Hydrogenated oils counterfeit natural saturated fat's solidity and spreadability similar to butter, the real thing, but much cheaper.[1] When pressurized hydrogen is added to vegetable oil, the artificially hardened product has good spreadability, greatly extended shelf life, and the product produces moist baked goods and other desired qualities.

Ubiquitous partially hydrogenated fats are used to manufacture thousands of common non-foods: stick margarines, chips, packaged microwave popcorn, icing, baked goods such as cookies, crackers, pies, cakes, snacks, ice cream, and many other non-foods; deep fried foods such as chicken nuggets, battered shrimp, donuts, and French fries."

This factory fat is found in foods in restaurants and fast food establishments. It is used for deep-frying. You've no doubt seen the piles of curly fries at state fairs. I have found some health food store products are made with TFA. These are "man-factured" products our bodies were not designed to process.

If the package ingredients include "partially hydrogenated," "shortening," or "mono-diglycerides," it is hydrogenated. The latter is called mono-diglycerides because it has a high monosaturated fat content. However, it is hydrogenated before it is separated out. Since we use only a few packaged foods, e.g., unrefined, non-hydrogenated extra virgin olive oil, unrefined, non-hydrogenated virgin coconut butter, and butter, we don't see these ingredients.

The FDA Food Advisory Committee voted in 2004 to recommend trans fatty acid intake be reduced to "less than 1% of energy (2 grams per day of a 2000 kcal diet)." To my way of thinking, no amount of toxins are safe to eat. trans fats simply are not in our diet.

---

[1] Fats are solid at room temperature. Oils are liquid at room temperature. Olive oil becomes solid in the refrigerator. All are lipids.

Two years later and effective January 1, 2006, all packaged food products were required to list trans fats on the Nutrition Facts panel. The amount of trans fats per serving of food must appear under the Total Fat section of the label *if* there is more than .5 grams. If you don't see trans fats on the label, you may total the values for saturated, polyunsaturated and monounsaturated fats. The total should equal "Total Fats." If it doesn't, the difference is trans fat.

"Zero grams trans fat" means less than .5 grams *per serving*, but "zero percent trans fat" means less than .5% of a 2,000 calorie diet (10 calories, or 1 gram per serving). Regardless, it depends upon the serving size and how many know how many grams are in half a cup?

What Did They Know & When Did They Know It?

One of the worst issues with the PD baggage is these trans fats (TFA) in vegetable oils it promotes. TFA are chemically defined as *un*saturated fatty acids, but are classified uniquely and separately from other fats because they are like no other fat. They are not biologically equivalent even to other *un*saturated fatty acids, do not function as essential fatty acids (EFA) as do other vegetable oils, and behave very differently than natural saturated fatty acids.

A 1989 Harvard Department of Nutrition study states, "Concern that trans-fatty acids [TFA] formed in the partial hydrogenation of vegetable oils may increase the risk of coronary disease, **has existed for several decades**..."

Dietary intake of TFA was found to be "...**directly related to risk of myocardial infarction**...Intake of margarine – the major source of trans-isomers – was significantly associated with risk of myocardial infarction."[1]

This study was performed nearly 20 years ago, and "concern" existed 30 years before it was published. Remember the distinguished members of the 1956 AHA fund raiser panel who delivered the lipid hypothesis and PD to the nation? Before that organization issued its first dietary guidelines, medical doctors

---

[1] Ascherio A, Hennekens CH, *et al*, Trans-fatty acids intake and risk of myocardial infarction, Harvard Dept. of Ntr, Jan. 1994 Jan;89(1):94-101

Page and Stamler, and researcher Keys, had published their papers stating that the increase in coronary heart disease (CHD) was "paralleled by increasing consumption of vegetable oils."[1]

The same year as the televised performance, Keys had "suggested that the increasing use of hydrogenated vegetable oils might be the underlying cause of the CHD epidemic."[2] Some of the medics wrote promo booklets sponsored by food oil companies; though in the beginning the American Medical Association opposed the commercialization of the lipid hypothesis. It even warned that "...the anti-fat, anti-cholesterol fad is not just foolish and futile... it also carries some risk," (the understatement of the ages).

How many *millions* of deaths and what incredible suffering and cost might have been prevented had the AMA prevailed, and the government acted at least at that time if not before, to put a halt to that "foolish and futile risk"? And yet masses globally are eating these death-dolling substances today.

Almost 25 years ago, when MI deaths in the US had soared to an alarming rate of 600,000 annually, the American researcher whom we mentioned earlier, Wayne Martin, completed his study review. He then confronted America's medics collectively for accepting the lipid hypothesis, and blaming saturated fats for the nation's disgraceful CVD level. Martin noted that human atheroma is composed mostly of fibers, fibrin, and dead cells, with but little cholesterol. He continued:

> "...It is suggested that MI is largely caused by coronary blood clots...that the introduction [in 1920] of a new, unnatural dietary fatty acid – trans-trans linoleic acid...caused vasoconstriction, while the clumping of platelets was greatly increased, giving rise to the coronary blood clots that either cause or are part of the fatal process of MI. It is suggested that in fostering the increase of dietary trans-trans linoleic acid in polyunsaturated

---

[1] For the detailed story, see Fallon's & Enig's, The Oiling of America, westonaprice.org/knowyourfats/oiling.html
[2] Keys A, Diet and Development of Coronary Heart Disease, *J Chron Dis*, Oct 1956, 4(4):364-380

vegetable fats at the expense of saturated animal fat, **orthodox medicine is fostering a principle cause of MI as the cure** [1] [emphasis supplied].

"Doctors out there are trying to get patients well. Medical organizations provide them with information they believe to be true...they rely on information that...is hopelessly outdated or biased,"[2] writes Dr. Bruce West. Yet these studies, performed at the nations best medical schools, are available to all, doctors and patients alike, and readily viewed on the Internet. Furthermore, researchers are gracious in their willingness to discuss their studies, to answer questions about them. Contact info is provided with the studies on the Internet.

Yet conventional medicine and nutrition, the media, and most all the related literature, refer to animal saturated fats and trans fatty acids (TFA) in the same breath; "...though TFA is worse," they say.

These are not comparable. About the only things the Creator's saturated fats and TFA have in common are the solidity and the general classification of "fats."

What Else Is Not Good About Trans Fats?

Harvard researchers found this partially hydrogenated vegetable oil increases LDL ("bad" cholesterol), and decreases "good" cholesterol (HDL); the more trans fat, the lower the HDL. (Saturated fat has the opposite effect, according to the previously mentioned studies.) Additionally, TFA increases triglycerides, causes "sticky" platelets and blood clots leading to heart attacks and strokes, based on other studies and highly respected Internet sources). When this fat becomes part of the cell membrane, it doesn't function as such, but allows the "bad guys" in while keeping the "good guys" out.

Partially hydrogenated soybean oil is related to "...ever-

---

[1] Martin W, The combined role of atheroma, cholesterol, platelets, the endothelium and fibrin in heart attacks and strokes. Med Hypoth, 1984 Nov;15(3):305-22

[2] West B, *Health Alert,* Sept. 2006, Vol. 23, Iss. 9

increasing rates of cancer, heart disease, infertility, impotence, asthma, allergies, learning disabilities, bone problems, digestive disorders, diabetes and obesity," warns Enig.[1]

Trans fat also increases unhealthy Lp(a) cholesterol, and reduces the particle size of this lipoprotein that compositionally resembles LDL. These small particles may become lodged between the endothelium (lining) and smooth muscles of arteries; then oxidize, become rancid, and inflame the lining, causing plaque formation and clogging arteries, leading to MI. We have long and often been advised to reduce saturated fat intake; but what about tampered-with oils? Only recently have we been alerted to the risk of even TFA.

Another Harvard study pointed to recent evidence that TFA increases *systemic* (not just localized) inflammation in the body, now considered to be a high risk factor for coronary heart disease (CHD). Inflammation is also directly linked to cancer.[2] Triggered by trans fats, inflammatory enzymes also "...eat away at joint tissue, they create bone-on-bone contact and the teeth-gritting pain that goes with it," says M. Cutler, MD.[3]

If we study the scientific literature regarding TFA, we may arrive at the conclusion that the decades of promoting the mixture that is the PD - which is enabled and upheld by the food industry - has produced precisely *that for which saturated fats have been blamed!*

What About Dr. Joliffe's Diabetes?

Trans fats have been linked to diabetes II. Dr. Joliffe suffered diabetes and its vascular thrombi (clots). In fact, cardiovascular disease is a major complication of diabetes II. Do you suppose that in the end this very unfortunate doctor might have considered that the Prudent Diet he religiously followed and strongly promoted – the "basket" into which he placed all his "eggs - may have been instrumental in his suffering diabetes, putting him at very high risk

---

[1] Enig M, The Tragic Legacy of Center for Science in the Public Interest (CSPI), westonaprice.org/knowyourfats/
[2] *Cell*, Jan. 26, 2007 (UC), also *Amer Jnl of Clin Nutr (*AJCN)
[3] Cutler, M, *Easy Health Options*, AL, 1/07

for vascular thrombi, and MI (he died before that happened) as well? Yet his was not counted as one of the deaths though he may have been perhaps the first to fall during that study.

The Profoundly High Costs To The Nation

American's continue dying from CVD at the rate of approximately nearly **one million annually,** or 2,740 *every day*.[1] That is the equivalent of 114 dying each and every hour of the day. Studies show that most of these deaths are associated with diet, plus resulting obesity, and lack of exercise. Would Americans tolerate **eight jumbo jets crashing** *every* **day with 350 passengers on board each, and all on board killed?** Yet we are doing just that in equivalent deaths. What if millions more were suffering terribly for years after a plane crash, before death? If this analogy seems extreme, it is actually understated. It is not possible to calculate the nation's costs of countless kinds, after approximately 75 years of rejecting the Creator's nutrition plan.

For more than 50 years we have been advised against God's good fats, which when eaten in moderate amounts, will satisfy, protect the heart, balance blood lipids, and oppose cancer. Yet foods rendered unrecognizable and often incapable of sustaining life, are offered to our uninformed, misinformed, malnourished masses.[2]

Approximately 64 million Americans are suffering heart disease, stroke and hypertension. Millions more are disabled. In 2004, the total direct economic cost of cardiovascular diseases in the U.S. was estimated to be **$368.4 billion.**[3] The indirect costs of adverse drug reactions (ADR) for 1997 are also unfathomable: 116 million *extra* physicians' visits, 76 million *extra* prescriptions, 17 million emergency room visits, 8 million hospital admissions, almost **200,000 deaths**, and nearly $77 **billion** in *extra* costs.[4] This is only extra cost for ADR's from properly prescribed drugs for the

---

[1] The low-fat diet did not change the death toll from CVD; carbs are still high.
[2] While this book concerns itself with America, the consequences of rejecting God's plan for eating are true for the globe, especially wherever altered foods are being consumed.
[3] Heart Disease and Stroke Statistics 2004 Update, AHA
[4] Pizzorno J, *Integrative Medicine,* Vol. 6, Nr. 1, Feb/Mar 2007

medical standard of care. Adverse drug reactions are the fourth leading cause of death in America.

In 2006, the prestigious *New England Journal of Medicine* published a Meta Analysis by researchers who reviewed many trans fat studies published during just the last decade or so.[1] The researchers calculated that elimination of TFA alone could save **between 72,000 and 228,000 heart attacks and deaths from heart disease *annually* in this country**.

Considering the **almost one million Americans** dying annually from heart disease, and that perhaps nearly all of them are consuming the PD, I suspect even 228,000 deaths from trans fats is a conservative but nevertheless horrendous figure. The *PD and altered foods may be responsible for the loss of more lives than the combined total of soldiers killed in all the wars America has fought since the American Revolutionary War.* Add to that, foreign populations to whom we export these "faux-foods."

Who Is Responsible?

Completely outlawing TFA alone would be one of the fastest, simplest ways to ultimately save countless lives, trillions of dollars, and significantly increase longevity in this country and abroad. That the federal government still has not taken this action after many decades of mass destruction is utterly reprehensible. And it seems no one is seriously held accountable, or paying a cent to the patients suffering terribly, or to their grieving families, or to all the rest of us who don't eat the world's fare and rarely get sick, but share in the numerous associated costs of others' eating.

A few are bothered when it appears inadequate studies are performed for some pharmaceuticals, e.g., if liver studies are not done with particularly toxic drugs. Yet altered foods have been shown to put consumers at risk for serious health conditions for a century, and obviously are allowed into the food system without adequate investigation and scientific studies. Shortening is a glaring example.

---

[1] Meta-analysis is a statistical procedure for combining data from multiple studies.

Before 1911, candles were made from animal fats; then cheaper cottonseed oil was hydrogenated so that it remained hard at room temperature. When electric lighting put a damper on the candle market, the manufacturer began marketing this as "shortening," as food. No one imagined the incredibly negative impact to the health of hundreds of millions for almost a century before it was investigated more thoroughly.

Cigarette companies are beginning to be held accountable for related health and death issues, even though warnings are printed on the labels and most people are aware that smoking "may be injurious to your health." However, there are no such labels on foods most consumers assume are perfectly safe. Should not the manufacturer and government be called to task for what is now scientifically shown to be linked with incredible morbidity and mortality rates?

Shortenings are now advertised as trans fat free (contain less than .5 grams of TFA). Present ingredients include fully hydrogenated oil and small amounts of partially hydrogenated oil. But do we know that fully hydrogenated oil is safe?

This fat contains an artificial ingredient called interesterified fat (IF). Already a study shows IF increased volunteers' blood sugar by a whopping 20%, and lowered the good HDL cholesterol. The rise in blood sugar is problematic if it puts more consumers at risk for diabetes and other diseases.[1] Back in 1989, a study showed IF caused fat metabolism disturbance when fed to omnivorous rats, whose diet naturally includes fat.[2] Yet when herbivorous rabbits were fed saturated fat not natural to their diets, saturated fats were declared harmful to humans, and removed from some previously approved diets.

After at least a decade of study "alerts," the FDA, instead of outlawing TFA, has only recently and simply ruled, that food labels must include "trans fats" if foods contain more than 0.5 grams of it. For multiplied millions that is too little too late. It presumes Americans are knowledgeable about this. How many people read or understand labels at all? And how many different foods or second helpings per day, do they eat which contain TFA?

---

[1] News, Yahoo, Jan. 24, 2007 (Wickipedia)
[2] Zsinka, *et al,* Natl Ctr For Biotech Info, NIH, Nahrung 1989;33(4):383

No amount of this unhealthy substance is acceptable for my loved ones or me.

Americans eat a very high percentage of their meals in restaurants and delis. From the deep-fried main dish to the piecrust, plus bread and margarine, and counterfeit coffee "creamers," these meals may far exceed the allowed TFA amount that requires a label, not that a label itself in anyway lessens the consequences. Even so, have you seen such labels on menus?

But in the end, we are responsible for what we choose to put in our mouths. *We* are responsible to educate ourselves; with the Internet and much literature alone providing the truth about what we eat, is there any excuse for us if we are unwilling to invest the time after so many have worked so hard to provide it? Or to grow even an organic tomato plant? The Bible tells us we are stewards of our temples of the Holy Spirit and it's to Him we must give an account.

Blind Trust Versus Informed Choice

If one wishes to compete with the Creator's whole foods - to imitate for profit - discrediting the real thing is important. Thus natural saturated fats have been castigated since the first counterfeits began appearing on US grocery shelves nearly a century ago. Trusting the federal government to protect us from all evil, we opened our mouths wide.

> Giant oil, food, drug, and medical industries are engaged in the pursuit of money. For all of them, health is a secondary concern. The blindly trusting consumer bears the consequences of the business bottom line, with compromised health.[1]

Thus Udo Erasmus, internationally recognized authority on the subject of fats and oils, encourages us to educate ourselves in that which affects our health. We as consumers have a responsibility to learn about what we put in our mouths. I have

---

[1] Erasmas U, *Fats That Heal, Fats That Kill,* Alive Books, BC, Canada ,1995, p. 93

given you here, a great deal to "chew on." Additionally, you may benefit significantly from specific website URL's provided you here, as well as materials listed in the resources section of this book, some leading you to others sources of this knowledge.

My family's fats and oils are animal-based foods, minimally processed coconut butter, extra virgin olive oil, avocados, nuts, and seeds, plus a small amount of unrefined, assayed cod liver oil. Fats and oils in general will be discussed along with carbohydrates in another book about that part of God's plan for eating after Eden.

Too Little Too Late?

If a serial killer was continually murdering even a few victims per year and the police were not aggressively pursuing the killer, there would be great outrage and a very loud outcry from the public. Yet here, we are talking about millions of lives and inestimable suffering and costs over the decades, and continuing. And what is our entrusted government doing about *stopping* it? Not enough.

It is not too late to stop stripping, devitalizing and toxifying our foods. Yet as the government continues to cave in to powerful interests that profit handsomely from production and sales of unhealthy substances we *choose* to put in our mouths, it is frustrating to consider the historical, cumulative effects, without more effective, protective regulation for the citizenry. But there *are* other ways....

First and foremost, Dr. Mozaffarian advises, "...The wisest thing is to eliminate anything made [with] partially hydrogenated oils." Anyone can immediately, proactively, protect himself or herself thus.

Years ago our son flew home for my 60th birthday weekend celebration at a wooded resort. On the way home we drove past a fast foods restaurant. He was very surprised when I said I wasn't sure but what the TFA might kill one faster than would cigarettes. There may now be studies to show that.

Yet who would have thought some of these establishments would act sooner than the government to discontinue their use of TFA! After all, before being pressured to switch to highly processed polyunsaturates for cooking, they had used stable beef tallow that is not damaged by reasonably high cooking temperatures.

It isn't because of the goodness of their hearts these and a few other establishments are no longer selling TFA foods. Even a little educating of the public about this toxin has made it more profitable for fast food corporations to take that action. It may be too early to know if their new deep-frying oils used about six days are healthy, though likely more so than TFA oils. However, there are other reasons not to eat deep-fried foods cooked to high temperatures in oils that are previously processed at high temperatures.

Denmark has already outlawed TFA. In the absence of US federal action to heed Dr. Mozaffarian's sagacious advice, major American cities are now considering this protection. New York City will soon outlaw TFA in restaurants.

An outcry from an educated populace is imperative and will speed the progress along. It seems that "voting with our dollars" may be quicker and more effective than waiting for the government.

At last, *one* of the worst food toxins is beginning to be exposed at a meaningful level in this country. Finally, backed by irrefutable, scientific study results, we consumers are beginning to be heard. May this increase exponentially.

Unsaturated Oils: A Reminder

From the abundant evidence, we can only conclude there are good reasons to be concerned, not only about partially hydrogenated and hydrogenated fats, but also regarding many vegetable oils being consumed.

A top researcher notes there is a small amount of even more toxic TFA in vegetable oils.[1] Likewise, when Dr. Enig analyzed USDA data of the McGovern Committee, she found that "…use of vegetable oils seemed to predispose to cancer; and animal fats, seemed to protect against cancer."[2] We also saw that Ray Peat, PhD, finds that such oils seriously interfere with the thyroid, "…and thus are likely to raise cholesterol."

---

[1] Dr. Mozaffarian in a personal email 3/07
[2] *The Oiling of America, Ibid.*

The Mozaffarian study discussed in this chapter included just one harmful effect of a steady diet of high carbs, especially refined ones. Most of those products will never be removed from the market. Therefore it is imperative that we help to educate those who wish to make informed choices for enhanced wellness.

The description of the processing of vegetable oils in Erasmus' book, *Fats That Heal, Fats That Kill,* also provides acrid food for thought. Enig's *Know Your Fats* and the abundance of such information at the Weston A. Price Foundation's website, are outstanding educational tools.

What if the government suddenly pulled all FTA and other vegetable oil products off the grocers' shelves? Perhaps one reason for not doing so is that the PD, the usual Americans diet, includes so many foods with these fats and oils the nation could not eat without radically changing their diets. Very few are that committed to wellness, thus the government tells us simply to try to reduce our level of dietary intake. Also, if the government ordered all TFA products discontinued or produced with safe saturates, the food industry might be shut down.

The Safest & Healthiest Way

> Consuming partially hydrogenated oils is like inhaling cigarette smoke. They will kill you -- slowly, over time, but as surely as you breathe. And in the meantime, they will make you fat![1]

The safest and healthiest way as always, is to consume the Creator's fresh, nutrient-dense foods, usually located in the perimeters of food stores. These are those (especially organically grown) that provide the body what it must have for continual healing, and in no way hinders that work, while sustaining optimum health.

---

[1] Eric Armstrong, TreeLight.com

5

It's In The Beef

With the exception of butter, no other food has been subjected to such intense demonization in recent years as red meat, particularly beef...Beef causes heart disease, say the Diet Dictocrats. Beef causes cancer, particularly colon cancer...[1]

CLA: Beef's Built-In Colon Protector?

Reliable studies show that red meat and whole milk may provide powerful properties that actually inhibit colorectal cancer (CRC), a leading cause of cancer-related deaths in the nation. One of these substances, conjugated lenoleic acid (CLA), is an *un*saturated fatty acid found only in red meat, whole milk (cow and goat), and whole milk derivatives. Rather than in the visible fat covering organs and seen around muscles, CLA is found in interstitial, non-visible fat in the meat.

In an Argentinian study, lean beef did not produce colon cancer. Rather the study showed large numbers of cancers being significantly reduced in a group of rats. Grass-fed beef with less than 15% saturated fat, appears to provide a ratio of CLA that is double that of high-fat meat. In this study, the meat became "protective of the colon" as in Bible times, and in some countries today. Its CLA also "promoted cardiovascular **protection against atherosclerosis.**"[2] A growing body of evidence shows that it

---

[1] Fallon S, Enig M, It's the Beef, westonaprice.org/mythstruths/mtbeef.html
[2] Grass-fed beef was not the source of the saturated fats participants consumed in the Mozaffarian study.

reduces the incidence, progression, and numbers of metastases and tumors of many kinds.[1]

The National Academy of Sciences announced in 1966 that CLA is "the only fatty acid shown unequivocally to inhibit carcinogenesis in experimental animals,...exhibiting consistent antitumor properties...even at very low levels..."[2,3]

The CLA appears to protect us by a mechanism of strong antioxidant activities against lipid (fat) peroxidation. As a scavenger for organic free radicals, CLA prevents tissue damage. Death of cancer cells (apoptosis) occurs when red meats and milk fats containing it, are consumed. In the lab (*in vitro*) CLA demonstrates cytotoxicity to malignant melanoma, breast, lung, and colorectal cell lines.[4] It is harmless to other cells. Thus consuming such red meat and milk fat products "...may produce a natural chemopreventative effect, without the additional cost of oral supplements or the need for disturbing dietary changes." [5]

Colon cancer and others, have been associated with obesity. Decreasing body fat storage, as CLA has been demonstrated to do, may be one of its antitumoral effects.

Milk fat has other anticarcinogens such as butyric acid, sphingomyelin, ether lipids, and metabolites of tumor suppressor lipids. Such properties may all work together (synergistically) with CLA, and along with the very important other nutrients and factors of milk and milk fat. (I have seen no studies regarding CLA in ultrapasteuized foods specifically.)

This Divine "additive" reduces blood cholesterol (hypolipidemic), is antioxidative, and is an antiatherosclerotic

---

[1] Eynard AR, Lopez, CB, Conjugated linoleic acid (CLA) versus saturated fats/cholesterol: their proportion in fatty and lean meats may affect the risk of developing colon cancer, Lipids in Health & Disease 2003, 2:6, doi:10.1186/1476-511X-2-6, Inst. De Biologia Celular, Catedra de Histologia, FCM-UNC/CONICET, Argentina

[2] Eynard, *Ibid.*

[3] Natl Rsrch Cncl (NRC): Carcinogens and anticarcinogens in human diet. 1996

[4] Parodi PW, Cow's milk fat components as potential anticarcinogenic agents, J Nutr 1997, 127:1055-1060

[5] Parodi PW, Eynard AR, Potential of essential fatty acids as natural therapeutic products for human tumors.
J Nutr 2003, 19:386-388.

nutrition (decreases risk of CVD) – without adverse effects.[1]

Contrary to much American conventional, nutritional hype, and properly processed, biblically grown and properly prepared, these foods may be recommended as "fitting well in a healthy diet."

A word of caution may be in order here. At least one study shows increased risk of CRC when meat was roasted too long. Other studies also show that toxic acrylamides, which also may cause cancer, are introduced with overcooking, as well as grilling and deep-frying.[2]

God's Whole Menu

With an unproven premise that red meat causes colon cancer, and admitting "...[it] does not promote cancer in rodents;" rats on a low calcium, 5% safflower oil diet, when fed hemin (not meat) from red blood cells, developed colon cancer in one study.[3] It was presumed that the hemin (representing red meat) was the culprit. Regardless of the many issues with the study, calcium, olive oil (replacing the vegetable oil, itself suspect), and antioxidants, inhibited the cancer in rodents.

There are great differences in whole, red meat and hemin supplementation. However, it is worth noting that God's whole menu as found in Scripture, includes good sources of calcium,[4] extra virgin olive oil, and antioxidants.

---

[1] Pfeuffer M, Schrezenmeir J, Bioactive substances in milk with properties decreasing risk of cardiovascular disease, Br J Nutr 2000, Suppl 1:S155-159

[2] The state of CA has sued major fast-foods companies for failing to warn consumers of the "use of a possibly toxic ingred." The state estimated French fries and potato chips contain as much as **125 and 75** times more acrylamides than requires a warning under present regulations. Answers.com. Jan. 2007

[3] Fabrice P, *et al,* Meat and cancer: haemoglobin and haemin in a low-calcium diet promote colorectal carcinogenesis at the aberrant crypt stage in rats; carcin.oxfordjournals.org/cgi/content/full/24/10/1683

[4] Abraham served his divine Guests milk (calcium source) with read meat. Gen. 18:5-9

Cholesterol – Do We Need It?

Cholesterol – the mere mention of it strikes near-terror in Americans' hearts – yet it is important to our health and survival. Contrary to conventional conviction, the healthy human body is unable to produce all its requirement for cholesterol. Why would God command His people to eat foods with saturated fats if they were not needed, even harmful?[1]

Discovered in 1784, "cholesterol" comes from the Greek *chole* (bile) and *stereos* (solid), plus the chemical suffix *–ol* from alcohol, though it does not act like alcohol. Your liver, brain, and spinal cord, possess high concentrations of this soft, waxy, waterproof substance. It is critical for cellular protection from chemical changes outside the cells; and for their optimal functioning, especially of nerve cells, and thus nerves themselves.

The liver normally produces 75-85% of cholesterol - approximately 1,000 mg. of cholesterol per day. Cholesterol is required for supporting the immune system,[2] healthy bones,[3] fluidity determination and waterproofing of cell membranes; feeding and protecting the heart[4] and liver;[5] as fuel for the cells' mitochondria (minute "power plants"); and utilization of essential fatty acids. Adequate amounts of cholesterol are *vital* for optimum health.

Cholesterol also plays a major role in the manufacture of bile, required for emulsifying and utilization of fats. It is important for the metabolism of fat-soluble vitamins A, D, E and K, and for bodily production of vitamin D. Thus it is also important for healthy bones.

Cholesterol, whether manufactured in the body or as dietary intake, is the chief precursor for your steroid hormones, cortisol

---

[1] We are not recommending eating cover fat and fat you can see when you eat your roast, steaks, or ribs. God says that fat belongs to Him (Lev. 3:16). Neither do we recommend consuming excess amounts of any food.
[2] Kabara, JJ, *The Pharmacological Effects of Lipids,* American Oil Chem. Soc., 1978-1-14
[3] Watkins, BA & Seifert, MF, *Food Lipids and Bone Health,* IN:IFT Basic Symposium Series.
[4] Lawson, LD, Kummerow, F, *Lipids,* 1979:14:501-503
[5] Cha, YS & Sachan, DS, *J Am Coll Nutr,* 1994, Aug.

and corticosterone; and aldosterone in the adrenals (helping us deal with stress and protecting against cancer and heart disease), as well as the sex hormones, and those derivatives.

Recently scientists have found cholesterol to be involved in cell signaling. More than one study shows saturated fats' protection against viral and other microbial damage.

Due to its stability - and unlike polyunsaturated vegetable oils - beef's saturated fat does not use your body's antioxidants, leaving your body vulnerable to increased cancer risk.

My family – with its very different genomes and metabolisms – has always eaten liberal amounts of fat sources, including animal-based foods, unrefined coconut butter, avocados, nuts, seeds, and extra virgin olive oil. For decades, upon presenting ourselves for annual physicals, our internist pronounced our blood fats to be "perfect" with "low CVD risk." Yet, blood cholesterol tends to decrease as old age approaches; and we would have preferred higher levels going into it.

The Lower The Better? Not!

"There is no certain correlation between serum cholesterol and coronary artery disease," declared the famous heart surgeon, Michael DeBakey, and his 1964 study with 1,700 participants.[1] At the same time, my sister, an open-heart surgical nurse, observed that most of those patients did not have high cholesterol. In fact, *most heart disease patients don't have higher cholesterol levels than those who do not develop heart disease*, according to experts.[2] Yet cholesterol is still the "step child" condemned countless times per day by conventional wisdom.

Not only does dietary fat *not* cause cardiovascular (CVD) disease, but *low* serum cholesterol may be the *real* culprit,[3] according to independent researcher, Professor U. Ravnskov, MD,

---

[1] DeBakey, M, *et al*, Serum cholesterol values in patients treated surgically for atherosclerosis, JAMA, 1964, 189:9:655-59

[2] Superko, HR, Inherited disorders contributing to coronary heart disease; Chol, Genetics, & Heart Dis Inst, 1996

[3] Ravnskov U; The retreat of the diet-heart hypothesis; *J. of Amer. Phys. & Surgeons* 8, No. 3, 2003:94-95; *O J Med* 95, 2002:397-403, Is atherosclerosis caused by high cholesterol?

PhD, who authored the book, *The Cholesterol Myths, Exposing The Fallacy That Saturated Fat And Cholesterol Cause Heart Attack,* and directed many timely studies.

Dr. Ravnskov also revealed that serum cholesterol is not a strong predictor of CVD.[1] In fact, high cholesterol is not predictive at all after the age of 47, according to the thirty year follow-up of the famous Framingham, Massachusetts population's heart study. Most surprising to many, "...those whose cholesterol went down had the highest risk of having a heart attack!" This two generation study, reported for each 1 mg/dl *drop* of cholesterol, there was an 11% *increase* in coronary and total mortality.[2] (Remember, low cholesterol combined with low albumin, is a strong predictor of mortality.)

Low serum cholesterol does not prolong life, and may signal high risks such as cancer, according to notable experts.[3] A patient treated at a veterans hospital, sued that agency for withholding his low total cholesterol (TC) figures from him in view of the countless studies he found demonstrating low cholesterol is associated with cancer.

What Are We To Believe?

The American Heart Association's (AHA) 1999 annual stroke conference revealed that cholesterol levels ***less* than 180 mg/dL doubled the risk of hemorrhagic stroke** compared to those with **cholesterol levels of 230 mg/dL**. Read it again!

Today, that website declares that serum cholesterol of 200-239 mg/dL is borderline risk, and high-risk serum cholesterol is anything over 240 mg/L. Previously it protected us from hemorrhagic stroke, now it seems 230 mg/dL is in the risky range.

To its great credit, the website of *Circulation,* journal of the AHA, includes countless studies from various medical journals with such subjects as "cholesterol-rich diets' usefulness with

---

[1] Ravnskov, U; *New cholesterol guidelines for converting healthy people into patients,* www.ravnskov.nu/uffe.htm

[2] Anderson KM, Castelli WP, Levi D, Cholesterol and mortality, 30 years of follow-up of the Framingham study, *JAMA,* 1987; 257:2176-2180

[3] Jacobs D, *et al,* Report of the Conference on Low Blood Cholesterol, AHA, *Circulation,* Vol 86, 1046-1060

tuberculosis [low cholesterol is common among these patients];" "immunoprotective effects of high cholesterol for atherosclerosis and infection," "cholesterol's association with cocaine addicts' relapse;" and many other important study extracts that the reader may find of interest.

An acquaintance told of his doctor's intention to get his patients' total cholesterol down first to 150, then to 100. "I aim to get mine down to zero!" the fellow crowed. "Normal cholesterol levels run around 150 to 250…cholesterol down around 80 to 130 – [is] a dangerous proposition for sure. It is at values around 100 or lower that people with serious deteriorating diseases and cancer succumb,"[1] advises Dr. Bruce West, who has successfully treated countless thousands of CVD patients.

And who knows where it will end? When you witness the cholesterol "bar" being lowered time after time, does it make you wonder if anyone really knows what is "high" or "low?" Again writes Dr. West:

> If it were up to most health professionals, we would eat no saturated fat, consume 6 to 10 servings of grain daily, keep blood pressure at 110/70 or less, and cholesterol at 150 or less with LDL less than 100. This prescription is impossible to follow, flies in the face of substantiated science, and would cause most people to wither as they slowly become diabetic.[2]

Low Cholesterol & Fetal Brain Damage

Severe birth defects have been linked to low cholesterol levels during the pregnancy. According to Professor Max Muenke, Director of Medical Genetics Branch of the National Human Genome Research Institute (US), speaking at the International Genetics conference in Melbourne, cholesterol deficiency in the pregnant mother may cause massive brain abnormality in the fetus.[3]

---

[1] West B, *Health Alert,* Sept. 2005, Vol. 22, Iss. 9
[2] *Ibid,* Sept. 2006, Vol. 23, Iss. 9
[3] *Sydney Morning Herald,* Severe Birth Defects Linked To Low Cholesterol Levels During Pregnancy, July 8, 2003 (journalist's name not supplied)

Most of these babies are spontaneously aborted early in the pregnancy, while 90% of the live births don't survive six months. The chief gene linked to HPE "...can only work properly when [this] protein is bound to cholesterol," explained Professor Muenke.

This is not a rare condition; rather it is *the* most common abnormality of the developing brain. The tragedy occurs in an astounding one of every 200-250 embryos lost in the US each year from this condition.

And In The Elderly...

Older people with high cholesterol have half the number of deaths from heart attacks as their peers with low cholesterol, according to a Yale University study.[1]

The position of *The Lancet,* the world's leading independent, general medical journal, is as follows:

> Our data accord with previous findings of increased mortality in elderly people with low serum cholesterol, and show that long-term persistence of low cholesterol actually increases the risk of death. Thus the earlier patients start to have lower cholesterol concentration, the greater the risk of death.[2]

According to an article carried in the *Canadian Medical Journal*, authored by E. Vos and cardiologist Colin P. Rose, lowering cholesterol in those over 70 years of age, may reduce coronary artery disease, however, there are offsetting incidents of cancer.[3] Low cholesterol, especially in older people (70-75 years of age), "...is a very, very bad finding."[4]

---

[1] Jnl. of the Amer Med Assn, 1994; 272:1335-40
[2] *The Lancet*, Vol. 358, Nr. 9279
[3] Vos E , Rose CP, CMAJ, Nov. 8, 2005; 173 (10).doi:10.1503/cmaj.1050120.
[4] West B, *Health Alert, Sept. 2005, vol. 22, Iss. 9*

The brain doesn't function as well without extra fat and cholesterol for seniors.[1] Studies also show that high total cholesterol (TC) in the elderly, reduces risk of dementia.

Low Cholesterol, High Suicide Rates

Depression, anxiety, and suicide are linked with low cholesterol, as reported in 1999 by the British Broadcasting Corporation (BBC), and confirmed by a recent South Korean study.

People in the lowest quartile of total cholesterol concentrations, have more than six times the risk of committing suicide, according to a study reported in The *Journal of Epidemiology*.[2] A famous example, Nathan Pritikin, MD, who gave us the low-fat diet, suffered from cancer and committed suicide. Low cholesterol is also associated with depression and cancer. Our internist says that all patients are now to be checked for depression.

I recall an old New York City study of autopsies of approximately 140 suicides, which revealed that 100% of them had low serum cholesterol.

Divine Diets For Farm Animals Too

God most often speaks to me upon awakening, before the busy day begins, and my mind is in gear. While writing this section, I was awakened about 4:30 one morning, got up and "happened" to open my Bible to Isaiah 30:24 where we are told that food animals are to be grass-fed, while work animals such as oxen and donkeys, requiring extra energy from carbs, are to be given grains as well.[3]

"Muzzle not the ox that grinds out the corn;" let these working animals partake of it, farmers are also instructed by their Creator.[4] Like many humans today eating excessive grains, grained animals

---

[1] Enig MG, *Know Your Fats,* Bethesda Press, 2001-190
[2] Ellison, *et al., Journal of Epidemiology,* 2001
[3] Winnowing refers to throwing grains into the air so that the wind blows the chaff away. It refers only to grains.
[4] Deut. 25:4

may accumulate excessive saturated fats unless they are work animals. Thus God told His people to feed only these animals high carb diets.

It's In The Beef

All foods that contain fats contain a variety of them. Saturated fat is not the only fat in animal-based foods; it's just the only one you hear about. About half the fat of beef is the monosaturated fat of heart-healthy extra virgin olive oil. Red meat also includes essential fatty acids (EFA) Omega 3 and 6. Ecosapenoic acid (EPA) is a heart-healthy fat also found in fish and cod liver oil, which makes platelets slippery, and is a blood thinner to prevent hypercoagulation.[1] Though unrefined Omega 6 is also important, Americans get far too much in processed foods, e.g. mayonnaise and salad dressings.[2] Most nutrition scientists find that we need less of it than Omega 3.

Richard Dewhurst, PhD, of the UK, wrote me about his recent studies of grass-fed beef cattle, having found that they have significantly higher Omega 3 (EPA) than Omega 6. The Omega 6 and Omega 3 ratio of grain-fed beef may be higher than 20:1, whereas grass-fed beef usually has a ratio of 0.16:1.[3] The grass-fed beef of the Bible was the latter.

Other studies show that feeding soy and grains to cattle causes reversal of the essential Omega 6 and Omega 3 (EPA) fatty acid ratios.[4] According to our local resources, even most beef sold by natural food stores, including organic, are grain-produced, giving likely fatty acid ratio similar to supermarket flesh foods. This is yet

---

[1] See also mercola.com/beef/omega3.htm regarding Omega 3 and pregnant and nursing women, and the need for EPA by infants. This nutrient may be obtained either by nursing mothers with adequate dietary EFA or from cod liver oil given infants and children.

[2] Fats other than saturated and trans fats, are discussed in *Eatin' After Eden – God's Whole Menu*.

[3] J. Anim. Sci. 2000. 78:2849-2855. See Chap. 5 concerning chickens fed soy and grain.

[4] And what might this combo do with human EFA ratios? (Our bodies need saturated dietary fat to utilize EFA.) Many chickens are also fed soy and grains; including all commercial layers, one such a manager told us.

another reason to promote and demand grass-fed beef, especially locally.

What to do? When local grass-fed beef is available, that is best; even if not organic. However, there are other reasons for purchasing the natural stores' meats when grass-fed is not an option. There are a number of Internet offerings as well. It is surprising how many resources become available when we are determined to obey the Word in our eating.

If it seems you have no good option, why not pray that God will provide one? He feeds the sparrows, and He is even more concerned with our food. Certainly we should pray over whatever we eat.

Some Additional Beef Benefits, Or "Meat Is Neat!"

An entire book could be written about the myths and plain misinformation disseminated about red meat. But this chapter is chiefly about what's *right* with God's nutritional gifts. And this gift is a superior source of nutrients. Besides all the essential amino acids and others for quality protein, plus good fats, there are the vital vitamins B_{12} and B_6, as well as magnesium and zinc.

Red meat is, in fact, a good source for vital healthy fats. Besides the monosaturated fat mentioned above, one-third of beef's saturated fat is stearic acid, shown not to raise blood cholesterol levels.

Surprising to even medical doctors and registered dieticians alike, studies have shown that beef works well in meal plans they use for decreasing blood cholesterol levels.

Research has shown that as much as six ounces on five or more days weekly, has no adverse effects. In fact, beef produces the same positive changes in blood cholesterol as white meat. In other words, healthy beef is as effective as skinless chicken for reducing blood cholesterol.

One of beefs full array of amino acids, carnitine, is important for a healthy heart.[1] Back in 1991, Chaitow foresaw also the

---

[1] Carnitine is produced in the human liver with adequate vit. C and lysine. To those people genetically unable to convert methionine or lysine, it becomes almost an essential amno acid, Bland suggested.

clinical use of carnitine with obesity since it enhances fat mobilization in the body.

With its "profound involvement" in fat metabolism and triglyceride reduction,[1]

> [Carnitine] is of potential value in conditions as diverse as intermittant claudication; poor circulation; myocardial infarctions, and kidney disease. Carnitine transfers fatty acids across the membranes of the mitochondria ["powerhouses" of the cells], where they can be utilized as sources of energy.[2]

Unfortunately, organ meats, very nutrition dense, are little enjoyed in America anymore. God's ancients and your grandparents included them in their diets to their great benefit. We are still able to get liver and heart with grass-fed beef.

Don't Leave Out Lamb![3]

We also buy local spring lamb for the freezer. Like other animal-based foods, this one is nutrient-dense, absolutely packed with essential nutrients for optimal health. It is rich in B vitamins; of course vital vitamin B_{12}; and others, including niacin for relaxing and getting to sleep, reducing harmful serum cholesterol levels while elevating "good" cholesterol and balancing the ratio; and reducing anxiety and depression. Like other B vitamins, niacin is water-soluble and must be provided daily. Just a three-ounce serving of lamb supplies the daily requirement for this nutrient.

Lamb is also high in iron (two times more than chicken or pork, and six times more than fish) for required for oxygen energy in muscles; and for brain functions of concentration and memory; zinc for the immune system, and of course, quality protein.

---

[1] Chaitow, L, *Thorson's Guide To Amino Acids*, 1991-72
[2] *Ibid.*, L, *Amino Acids In Therapy, A Guide to the Therapeutic Application of Protein Constituents*, Healing Arts Press, VT, 1988-76
[3] USDA, 1999 Nutr. Database for Standard Reference, Supp. Data on Australian Lamb, pp. 147-246

Forty percent of lamb fat is monounsaturated, the same as found in olive oil. One three ounce serving of lamb includes only five grams of fat. Usually lamb is grown on green, lush pasture in the spring.

What About The Fat?

Invisible fat within the muscle is healthy as we have explained. Other fat is to be trimmed away. Leviticus 3:17 commands us not to eat the fat (cover of muscle and organs) or blood:

> And it shall be a perpetual statute for your generations throughout all your dwellings, that ye eat neither fat nor blood.

Our Lungs Need Saturated Fat

In her book, *Know Your Fats: The Complete Primer for Understanding the Nutrition of Fats, Oils, and Cholesterol,*[1] Mary Enig, PhD, explains that our very important lung surfactant, is a special phospholipid with 100 percent saturated fatty acids, 68% of which is palmitic acid."[2] (Non-hydrogenated palm oil is 45% palmitic acid; butter and chicken fat are approximately 25% palmitic acid.) America's PD is woefully lacking in this nutritional support for healthy lungs.

What do you suppose might be another effect of a diet without adequate, quality, saturated fat? Could it contribute to the rising incidence of cancer and other lung issues? "...[W]hile smoking was widespread at the turn of the century, myocardial infarction was not. This suggests that there may be factors in traditional diets that protect against the negative effects of smoking," wrote Enig and Fallon.[3]

---

[1] Bethesda Press, MD, 2000
[2] Enig, M, Food, Farming, and the Healing Arts, *Wise Traditions*, 2000, Summer
[3] Fallon S, Enig M, "What Causes Heart Disease?" *Wise Traditions* , Weston A. Price Foundation

6

Eggs: God's Amazing "Gold Standard"

"Nature's Perfect Food"

Nutritionists worldwide rate all protein foods in comparison to the egg. Why? Because the humble egg is the most perfect protein food known to mankind.

How did they determine this? The quality of protein foods is first rated by how many kinds of essential amino acids (EAA) are found in each; and whether each is complete or incomplete protein. Animal-based protein foods have all EAA in a single source. With these protein building blocks, the greater their quantity, the higher the quality of the protein food.

Now that you know that animal-based (meat) protein is the highest quality of protein - and the body's first choice for this macronutrient – you do not need to remember which foods have complete protein.

Just as a reminder, a food protein is considered complete if it has all the essential amino acids. However, our bodies require amino acids in certain proportions. If one or more are low, those amino acids are called limiting amino acids, and our bodies cannot use all the amino acids completely.

Nutrition scientists classify protein foods by assigning them a chemical value based on how well they match the exact pattern of amino acids needed for protein synthesis within the human body. Eggs, "nature's perfect food," merit a 100% rating, the highest of any food.

Having said that, I must be quick to add that we are not what we eat, but what we eat, digest, and utilize. Enzymes must split up the large protein molecules into separate amino acids in order for protein digestion to be completed. Methods of cooking greatly influence this process.

When amino acids have been altered by prolonged or high heat, the protein is said to be denatured. Eggs also contain lecithin which emulsifies the fat in them.[1] However, if they are overly cooked, the lecithin is prevented from doing its work.

The Biological Utilization Rate For Eggs

Another measure of protein quality is the biological value (BV) rating. It measures the amount of protein (nitrogen) *retained* per gram *absorbed.* The more nitrogen excreted in fecal matter and urine, the less of a particular type of protein is utilized by cellular construction. A BV of 100 is the highest utilization humanly possible, meaning that 100% of the protein (nitrogen) was used, and none at all lost. (No more than one gram of nitrogen can be stored for each one gram of nitrogen consumed.) Eggs scored 100%.

Generally, this is the rate of efficiency with which protein is used by the body for growth, regeneration of muscles, skin, and all other body tissues, as well as immunity and for strength training. That includes our body's production of hormones, enzymes, and antibodies, vital to your health and survival.

Again, eggs rate higher than all else - twice as high as beans, with beef, salmon, and chicken in between.[2] No wonder nutrition scientists employ eggs as the standard of measuring the protein quality of other foods. Yet conventional nutrition often urges us to avoid them! Whether or not you have access to healthy meats, if farm-fresh eggs are available, partake of them liberally.

---

[1] To emulsify is to combine two liquids which normally would not mix easily. Lecithin (Grk. *Lekithos* meaning egg yolks) enables the suspension of cholesterol into minute droplets so that it can be transported in the blood to needy cells. Lecithin also helps maintain proper cholesterol level.

[2] Some claim that isolated whey rates 104; as exlained, that is impossible.

Growing On Eggs

The relationship of intake to growth is called the protein efficiency ratio. At 100, eggs are once again at the top. Considered "the gold standard" and a highly bioavailable, nutrient-dense food, eggs supply the highest nutrition of anything to be found in a supermarket, including those from caged hens. Egg protein, and the number of nutrients eggs contain, are the standard by which all others are compared.

Again, the quality is even more superior (both the meat and eggs) when hens are raised on green pasture, allowed free exercise in the sunshine and fresh air, and can scratch for worms for their own protein, as the Creator intended. Alternating grassy plots on our farm, our happy hens sang sweetly even in the cold rainy winter. Observing their constant contentment in the worst weather and circumstances, one finds complaining out of place.

Besides providing an excellent source of highest quality protein, "hen fruit" (the egg) is obviously one of God's most nutritious foods. With a list of vitamins and minerals as long as your arm - about fifteen in all - these include vitamins B_{12}, D, zinc, and iron, in which vegetarians are often periously low. Actually, eggs have all the nutrients necessary to produce a whole, viable chick. That includes all the vitamins, minerals, trace minerals, carbohydrates, fats, and quality protein required for life. Eggs are simply nutrient-dense foods.

Eggs For The Eyes Of The Elderly

While the carotenoids lutein (loo-teen) and zeaxanthin (zee-ah-zan-thin), are found in other bodily tissues, they exist at 500 times more concentration in the macula of the eye, meaning the eyes have a strong need for them.

Except by the hand of the Great Physician, there is no cure or surgery for age-related macular degeneration (ARM). It is the leading cause of blindness in the aged. Therefore, prevention is critical. These nutrients have been "...strongly implicated as being protective against [ARM] and cataracts...," according to the USDA. They are found in easily eaten egg yolks.

Researcher Elizabeth Johnson, PhD, investigator in age-related eye diseases with the USDA Nutrition Human Research Center On Aging, arranged studies to determine blood serum levels of lutein from cooked spinach, eggs, and lutein supplements themselves. Each source provided 6 mg. of lutein/day. Dr. Johnson measured blood serum lutein concentrations from volunteers before and after testing. *Without exception,* the lutein levels were approximately 300% greater after eating eggs than after eating the same dosage of lutein from other sources.

Another recent study published in the *American Journal of Clinical Nutrition*, reveals that the carotenoids in egg yolks are better absorbed than those from carrots and other plants.

Cholesterol & Eggs: More Is Even Better?

Dr. Uffe Ravnskov, world renown researcher, personally tested the theory of eggs dangerously increasing cholesterol. He ate 59 eggs in 9 days! Instead of his blood cholesterol spiking, it acutally *fell* by more than 11%.

University of Conetticut researchers found that even three eggs per day do not increase heart disease risk factors in healthy older people.[1] Sometimes when eggs are added to the diets of those who have been afraid to eat them, the total cholesterol and "bad" LDL may rise a small amount, but there is a greater "good" cholesterol, HDL, increase.[2] In other words, the heart risk actually *decreases*.

This validation of God's nutrient-dense food, is very important because about half of all seniors quit eating eggs years ago for fear they would increase their cholesterol and heart disease risk. We know that cholesterol does not cause or increase heart risk, though it may point to an underlying issue, as Ravnskov proved.

Studies do not support the need for healthy seniors to restrict dietary cholesterol; instead, they need *more* cholesterol as they age. Especially do they need eggs, an affordable, nutritionally superior, chewable source of complete protein and many other nutrients.

---

[1] J. Of Nutr., Dec. 2005
[2] I have found the same when unrefined coconut butter is added to the diet.

Professionally and personally, it has long saddebed me that millions of older citizens have deprived themselves of that which they need for balanced nutrition and optimum health, because they have been misled by the misled and presumption!

"Many older individuals lack the nutritional balance that is required for optimal health because they are following inappropriate risk reduction interventions," Maria Luz Fernandez, PhD, declared. Egg substitutes, skim milk, skinless chicken, and others, are among the devitalized foods on which today's seniors subsist. Dr. Fernandez, who directed the UC study, advised that "Previous studies have not supported a need to restrict dietary cholesterol in healthy individuals aged 65 and over. Instead, such restrictions may cause nutritional shortfalls," she cautioned, and added that the UC study was conducted "…to see whether or not a dietary cholesterol challenge [three eggs/day] would affect any of three important measures of cardiovascular disease risk in healthy older people."[1] *It did not.*

Previous work by Dr. Fernandez, *et al*, produced similar results in healthy children, men between the ages of 20 and 50, and premenopausal women. (It did not include studies on diabetics [who have lipid issues] and pre-existing heart disease.)

Then why are patients being ordered by their medical doctors at wellness appointments, and advised by dieticians and conventional nutritionists on TV, radio, and in magazines, not to eat the Creator's wholesome and urgently needed foods, just as He created them to be eaten? Especially since as we age, absorption decreases and increased nutrition is increasingly vital.

The AHA has decided that 300 mg./day of dietary cholesterol is all that's allowed. A large egg contains only only one and one-half gram of saturated fat of the five grams of fatty acids it contains, not a meaningful amount. The other fats are monosaturated and polyunsaturated. However, these good fats are important for bodily hormone production, cell membranes, energy, and absorption of fat-soluble vitamins A, D, E and K they contain.

Not incidentally, eggs have thirty times as much real vitamin D as a full glass of reduced fat milk. No wonder Jesus referred to

---

[1] J. Of Nutri. Dec. 2005

them as "good gifts."[1] Luke 11:11-13 refers to eggs as "good gifts to your children."

Eggs are readily available even though healthy meat may be hard to find in some areas. You may even be able to keep a couple of hens for this great gift from God. Free range eggs are superior to other supermarket eggs, though I would prefer pastured hens' production if available. What is meant by "free range" and "pastured"? Here's how they're defined.

"Free Range" Versus "Pastured"

Range or free-range chickens are legally those who have certified access to the outdoors. We are told they may have as little as a foot or so space per each chicken. Small openings in the sheds may often restrict exiting, and the grounds may be surfaced with gravel, concrete, or whatever.

Pastured hens are raised just as it sounds – on grassy pasture. They obtain exercise while walking in the sunshine and scratching for earthworms and bugs that increase their nutrition and consequently their eggs' nutrients. This traditional method of caring for poultry is ecologically sustainable and humane. It produces the tastiest eggs from happy hens. I always found the "barnyard chorus" very peaceful and relaxing.

Like grass-fed beef's higher Omega 3 fatty acid, pastured hens' eggs (organic ones) provide up to 20 times more of the heart-healthy omega-3 (EPA), 35% less cholesterol, and 40% more vitamin A than other eggs. The Omega 3/Omega 6 ratio may be reversed in eggs of "factory hens" producing most supermarket eggs.

The best sources for pastured hens' eggs are local farmers where you see hens roaming the pasture rather than inside portable fences. These usually are raised without antibiotics in their feed, though are not necessarily organic. But even fed laying mash, their eggs may be superior to the usual supermarket eggs from caged hens. With high, dark yellow yolks and thick whites (albumin), these fresh eggs are a bargain at any price!

---

[1] Luke 11:11-13

Eggs And The Beauty Mineral

Eggs are the chief source of dietary sulfur Pfeiffer referred to as "the forgotten essential element."[1] Also known as "the beauty mineral," sulfur, is found in every cell of the body, especially the skin, hair, nails, and joints.

Just six nonmetallic elements account for 97% of the weight of most organisms, sulfur being one of them; along with oxygen, carbon, hydrogen, nitrogen, and phosphorus. Like the water soluble vitamins B and C, sulfur is not stored in the body and is constantly being used up and depleted without a regular source, such as eggs. Hence, sulfur is of dietary significance for good health.

Vegetarians and others are prone to sulfur deficiency, and especially so if they do not eat eggs. "Junk science" with its cholestrophobic warning against eggs, and "inappropriate risk reduction intervention," may account for a multitude being deficient in sulfur.[2] To hear some tell it, God should have placed a warning in the Word to restrict egg consumption to 2 or 3 weekly; or just not have created hens!

Ironically, eggs can be protective of the heart in a number of ways. About ten years after the PD was adopted, the American Cancer Society completed an eight-year retrospective survey of 800,428 people. Participants eating only five or more eggs a week, plus "a considerable amount of meat and greasy food had slightly fewer heart attacks and stroke deaths than those who ate fewer than five eggs a week and less of those other supposedly dangerous foods."[3]

Egg Safety

Conventional wisdom warns of salmonella poising from eating undercooked eggs. Is this a genuine risk or just another "urban

---

[1] Pfeiffer, CC, *Zinc and Other Micro-Nutrients,* Pivot Original Health Edition, 1978-74

[2] The high sulfur content of egg yolks is also helpful in normalizing intestinal flora after an antibiotic course.

[3] Hattersly JG, *Townsend Ltrs For Drs and Pts,* June 2002

legend" to convince us not to eat eggs? They also tell us to be sure and limit ourselves to just one egg, and to be sure to overcook it, thereby denaturing the protein and other nutrients.

I have never known of a case of egg-related bacterial infection. That doesn't mean there may not be any, but I suspect they are rare. However, the US Department of Agriculture (USDA) has found eggs to be a potential carrier of food-borne illness and recommends that infants, the elderly and immuno-compromised people avoid raw eggs. My medical adviser adds HIV, cancer, organ transplant patients, and children, to the USDA list of those who should avoid raw eggs. To be completely safe, don't eat raw eggs! The American Egg Board explains the risk thus:

> The inside of an egg was once considered almost sterile. But, over recent years, the bacterium *Salmonella enteritidis* (*Se*) has been found inside a small number of eggs. Scientists estimate that, on average across the U.S., only 1 of every 20,000 eggs might contain the bacteria. So, the likelihood that an egg might contain *Se* is **extremely** small – 0.005% **(five one-thousandths of one percent)**. At this rate, if you're an average consumer, you might encounter a contaminated egg once every 84 years.
>
> Bacteria, if they are present at all, are most likely to be in the white and will be unable to grow, mostly due to lack of nutrients. As the egg ages, however, the white thins and the yolk membrane weakens. This makes it possible for bacteria to reach the nutrient-dense yolk where they can grow over time **if** the egg is kept at warm temperatures. But, in a clean, uncracked, fresh shell egg, internal contamination occurs only rarely. [1]

Eggs lose weight quickly when stored uncovered in the refrigerator, where they should always be kept. If you purchase them in open-faced cartons that allow you to view them, when you get home, either place them in a closed container, or place a couple of layers of paper towels or some fabric over them.

---

[1] American Egg Board, Nov. 17, 2006

Needing Natural Nourishment *Now?*

Do you, or someone you know, need extra protein and nourishment beginning today? Even an extra egg per day can be beneficial for those with special nutritional needs. Growing children, older people who wish to prevent muscle loss; those with poor fitting dentures or anyone who finds chewing a chore; surgical patients and those with wounds; athletes in resistance training; and especially vegetarians – most all of us can benefit from the extra quality protein of eggs. An excellent way to enjoy eggs is to add a raw yolk from free running hens, to smoothies.

Milk & Eggs: The Divine Duo

High quality protein of raw dairy foods was consumed daily in Bible times.[1] Proverbs 27 instructed Jehovah's chosen people in the keeping of a utilitarian flock of goats, including verse 27 regarding milk:

> And thou shalt have goats' milk enough for thy food, for the food of thy household, and for the maintenance of thy maidens.

"Maintenance" in this verse speaks of a regular, continual supply of raw milk products - goat milk in particular - with their complete protein, carbs, saturated and unsaturated fats, important vitamins and minerals, and phytonutrients. Dr. Bernard Jensens book, *Goat Milk Magic*, explains in detail why fresh goat milk is superior when available. We find it especially good for making home-made icecream, with stevia. Not only in Bible times, but today World Vision explains the life-and-death value of goats:

> The early-morning bleating of a dairy goat is a happy sound for children in countries like Haiti and Kenya. They know it's ready to be milked! A goat nourishes a family with fresh milk, cheese, and yogurt, and can offer a much-needed income boost by providing offspring and extra

---

[1] To learn all about raw milk, go to www.realmilk.com

dairy products for sale at the market. It even provides fertilizer that can dramatically increase crop yields. A perennial favorite, both to give and receive![1]

Hens, chicks, eggs, and bird eggs for eating, are mentioned in the Bible. As we said, Jesus declared eggs good in Luke 11:12 and 13. Even the poor could keep one goat and a few chickens and enjoy quality, animal-based protein. Only eight ounces of milk and a couple of eggs supplies twenty grams of quality protein.

It Doesn't Hurt to Ask Him!

Years ago while experiencing allergic reactions with chicken eggs, I found I could well tolerate duck eggs. I located a source about five miles away when a couple of mallards nested in Donna's large back yard. All was well until one duck flew away and Donna couldn't locate the nest of the other.

I had so enjoyed and savoured each bite of the huge, creamy eggs. When I ate the last one I cried out to Father, "Oh God, I *need* this nutrition. *Please* find me some more duck eggs." About a couple of hours later Donna called back: "I found the nest and I have a *dozen* eggs for you!"

Jesus said if we ask for an egg, He will not give us something harmful; that is, eggs are good. No matter how loud and how often the conventional nay-sayers declare otherwise, I believe the One who created them. The evidence is ample!

Another Hearty, Healthy Breakfast

2-3 eggs over easy or lightly stirred, lightly scrambled
2 slices turkey bacon (do not cook until crisp)
Vegetables sauteed in EV olive oil or unrefined coconut butter
2 oz. buckwheat groats or spelt grains
1 cup beef or chicken homemade broth (see recipes on the Internet)

---

[1] As viewed Dec. 2006 at World Vision:
donate.wvus.org/OA_HTML/xxwvibeCCtpItmDspRte.jsp?section=10024&item=78&campaign=106634176&cmp=BAC-106634176

The two eggs and two slices of uncured, organic turkey bacon, supply twenty-two grams of complete protein, almost half the total amount needed for women for the day. It will maintain stable blood sugar, and facilitate functioning well in mid-afternoon without fatigue and sleepiness.[1] Shredded cheese may be substituted for the turkey bacon, or other meats.

As to carbs, if you prefer bread, eat one-half slice organic, sprouted spelt, other sprouted bread, or whole grain sour dough bread, warmed in a pan with butter or unrefined coconut butter. This provides approximately ten grams of complex carbohydrates for energy as you break your fast and some for later, plus good fat.

Buckwheat groats are much more nutritious than bread, and cook quickly on low heat. Presoaked whole spelt grain,[2] with butter and sea salt, is also excellent for breakfast or any meal. Both are more easily digested as a source of high carbs (eat no more than 1/3 cup) and additional complete protein.

Cultured, plain yogurt with stevia powder, is also a good source of low carbs . A glass of raw or pasteurized whole milk, especially goat milk, is also an excellent choice. If more protein is needed, easily made yogurt or fresh milk will supply one gram per ounce plus many other nutrients.

A Nourishing Breakfast "On The Run"

While an unhurried, sit-down meal is always best, sometimes schedules don't allow for that. But you need not go without a good day's start. A simple and nutritious smoothie can work well at such times. With my office in my home, and lunch as our main meal, I sometimes have a delicious smoothie for dinner. If more protein is desired, I add either goat milk powder or Smart Protein (whey).

---

[1] Caffeine addiction may cause a mid-afternoon slump if regular "fixes" are not forthcoming.
[2] Mellanby found that when there is adequate vit. D_3, the enzyme phosphatase breaks down the ca.-phytase chelate and releases ca. and also active phosporus for absorption.

Nothing Lacking Smoothie [1]

    8-10 oz. whole milk
    1 or 2 tsps. green powder or one from HFS
    ½ c. berries, fresh or frozen
    Stevia powder to taste
    1 scoop goat milk powder or whey protein powder

This quickie includes good amounts of macronutrients protein, carbs, and fats, and approximately 20 grams protein. The Springreen powder supplies many other nutrients without alfalfa with its phytoestrogen.

    It is not necessary to divide protein, carbohydrates, and fat equally between meals, though some protein should be eaten at each meal. It *is* important to pack plenty of protein into breakfast along with a little carbohydrate, and good fat.[2] The majority of carbs should then be eaten for lunch or dinner, depending upon what works for you. If you pack a lunch and find it easier to work with carbs for that meal, eat most of them then, with the balance of protein and low carb vegetables for dinner, or vice versa.

    If you are retired or otherwise able to eat your main meal at lunch time, so much the better. Regardless, breakfast should always contain quality, high protein of about 20-25 grams, and some protein should be eaten at every meal.

    Sprinkled with grated raw cheese, non-starchy vegetables are delicious over soft scrambled eggs. We enjoy chopped onion, bell pepper, and zucchini sauteed in a tablespoon or two of extra virgin olive oil, plus salt and pepper to taste. However, you should feel free to use whichever low-carb vegetables strike your fancy. Carbs in the evening help some people get to sleep.

---

[1] High vit. cod liver oil taken after the smoothie, with its vit. A, D & F, will help transport the milk ca.to the bones.

[2] Studying low carb nutrition on thousands of patients for forty years, Wolfgang Lutz, MD, found that 72 grams per day worked very well for them, divided among meals as they preferred.

Today's "Conventional" Breakfast

Contrast the nutrient-dense Hearty, Healthy Breakfast above with the typical, high carb (glucose spike), low nutrient, breakfast shown below. Which do you suppose will "stick to your ribs" after mid-morning, and prevent afternoon let-down, both of which may send one running for more refined carbs?

Low Protein - High Carb Spiker

1 glass orange juice	1 c. coffee
¾ c. dry, cold cereal	1 c. skim milk
1 banana or ½ cup berries	2 tsp. margarine
2 slices "whole wheat" toast	1 T. jelly or jam

This breakfast consists almost entirely of carbohydrate that will become glucose. It has triple the amount Lutz found to be so successful with his patients for nearly half a century.[1] Instead of seventy-two grams, the conventional total count for the day is approximately three hundred twenty-five whopping, fattening grams! Except for the "man-ufactured" margarine,[2] *all these foods require insulin to process,* guaranteeing a blood sugar spike and crash for many at mid morning, with need for an afternoon pick-me-up.[3]

To put it briefly here, carbs stimulate release of insulin that stores excess glucose as *saturated* fat in your body. No wonder America is struggling with overweight and morbid obesity.

The only meaningful amount of protein in this breakfast is about eight grams in the skim milk. Unfortunately it is likely ultrapasteurized so that the protein is denatured, and may be difficult to digest and assimilate. The nutritive value of the meal is comparatively low. You will learn more about carbs in my upcoming book.

---

[1] Allan, CB & Lutz, W, *Life Without Bread,* Keats Pub., 2000
[2] Any way you slice it, margarine cannot be compared with God's good, nutritious butter, especially raw butter.
[3] Coffee stimulates glucose release, indirectly also affecting insulin.

Very importantly, the mitochondria in your cells, your energy "power houses," are designed by the Creator, to use right fats for fuel. Here is an example of feedback I receive from patients who come to me consuming high carbs (especially at breakfast), low fats, and almost no animal-based foods.

Jim's Exciting Learning Experience

Seeking help with his diet for enhanced nutrition, this fifty-five year old professional came with skewed blood fats, especially low HDL (the "good" cholesterol), and at high risk for CVD, according to his physician. Besides teaching him the basics of good, whole-foods nutrition, I recommended some good nutrition teaching "tools" for this avid reader. We discussed his menus, sack lunches, and food preparation. Highly motivated, Jim soon switched to all organic foods, including a new garden that included five children's "help." They were soon playing hide and seek in and out and under the pole beans, which they harvested and helped cook, along with other "pickings" from the garden.

We added unrefined cod liver oil and coconut butter, plus a couple of whole foods concentrates. Having repeatedly reported how very good he now feels, Jim is also excited about his presently normal blood fats after only a short time of enjoying God's plan of mostly fresh foods.

I do not diagnose, prescribe, or treat patients. I simply taught Jim fresh, whole-foods nutrition, including principles of food selection. Much of it is contained in this and the next book. Jim replaced low-nutrient substances with real, nutritious food; listened to his body and observed the increasing levels of homeostasis as it began thriving with improved resources for its healing of itself, and growth.

This student's genome legacy includes heart disease from both mother and father. Teachable and highly motivated, he wants to avoid such at all cost for his young son's sake. Jim also exercises regularly, is at peace with God and his fellowman, spends much quality time with his family. Physician validated and monitored, the prospects are very good that he will reach old age without CVD or degenerative disease of any kind, as will his son, for whom he cooks.

After reporting the exciting, quickly improved test results of his blood fats, including HDL "good cholesterol" previously 34, now at 50 after about two months, triglycerides now 53, total cholesterol now 167 (studies show a little higher is healthier as he ages), with significantly improved coronary risk, plus fasting glucose of 80, and other healthy achievements, he continued:

> My MD...said to continue to adhere to the whole grain, LOW fat diet, etc. [high carb/low fat] I didn't tell him and I don't think he knew that my results were from adhering to the opposite of what he recommended! (and to think I went for over 20 years without eating eggs. I really like eggs!).

Jim had not told his medical doctor about his food choices and that he was working with a whole-foods nutritionist. I explained that his silence was not a good plan for any of us. His doctor needs to know what his patient is doing for himself nutritionally.

Since Jim's medical doctor advises his patients about nutrition and noted this patient's diet was working remarkably well, he would surely be interested to know what this is. With his dad's MI death, at age 54, Jim is motivated to educate himself and live healthfully.

What's Left?

If most animal-based foods, and fats, are eliminated from the diet, basically all that's left as the majority consume it, are chiefly carbs and non-foods. This may be profitable for the health care industry, but is it healthy for patients?

7

Why Not Soy Protein?[1]

The Comparison

A motor scooter may get one to work – if one ignores heat, rain, insects in one's eyes, or the risk of being run over. Yet it is not to be compared to a private luxury limousine, with plush upholstery, intercom, entertainment center, refrigerator, and a professional chauffer who assumes full responsibility for getting you there safely.

Neither should soy be compared with nutrient-dense, protective, animal-based vital foods we have discussed in this book. Though soy is high in protein, before you have completed your research, you may decide there might be risks associated in eating large amounts. Certainly the opinion of many researchers is that it does not compare with all that animal-source protein can do to improve and maintain optimum levels of wellness.

Yet as a multibillion-dollar industry, soy is one of the world's most powerful; it enjoys strong influence over the media, research institutions, and government agencies for starters. Though an impressive array of scientific evidence declares "soy is not a fit food for man nor beast,"[2] few individuals make the effort to investigate what they put in their mouths, often on a daily basis, including those who rely on this for their chief source of protein. Touted as "the miracle food that will feed the world," we should

---

[1] This chap. is dedicated to the memory of Valerie James, who valiantly and persistently fought against soy foods, including infant formula, for our benefit and for the generations to come. Valerie passed away Feb. 23, 2008. We share a link with the outstanding http://www.soyonlineservice.co.nz/

[2] True Health magazine, May/June 2004.

ask ourselves, "What are the short and long term effects of this controversial food?"

There are many excellent and bold means to educate you further regarding soy's benefits and its downside, as found in the Resources section of this book. The Weston A. Price Foundation's excellent educational website includes some listed below, followed by discussions of some other troubling ones everyone should learn about who consumes soy.

SOME SERIOUS CONCERNS WITH SOY[1]

A. High levels of phytic acid in soy reduce assimilation of calcium, magnesium, copper, iron and zinc. Phytic acid in soy is not neutralized by ordinary preparation methods such as soaking, sprouting and long, slow cooking.[2] High phytate diets have caused growth problems in children.[3]
B. Trypsin inhibitors in soy interfere with protein digestion and may cause pancreatic disorders. In test animals, soy-containing trypsin inhibitors also caused stunted growth.
C. Soy phytoestrogens 1.) disrupt endocrine function and have the potential to cause infertility, and to promote breast cancer in adult women; and 2.) are potent antithyroid agents that cause hypothyroidism and may cause thyroid cancer. In infants, consumption of soy formula has been linked to autoimmune thyroid disease.
D. Vitamin B_{12} analogs in soy are not absorbed and actually increase the body's requirement for B_{12}.
E. Soy foods increase the body's requirement for vitamin D.
F. Fragile proteins are denatured during high temperature processing to make soy protein isolate and textured vegetable protein. [Such] processing...results in the formation of toxic lysinoalanine and highly carcinogenic nitrosamines. Free glutamic acid or MSG, a potent neurotoxin, is formed during

---

[1] Used by permission from the foundation. WestonAPrice.org/soy/index.html.
[2] "Nor by the modern mass-production processes that are applied in everyday grocery items," says SoyOnLine Serv.
[3] Beginning with infant formula and other foods, America's chldren are getting large amounts of soy.

soy food processing, and additional amounts are added to many soy foods.

G. Soy foods contain high levels of aluminum, which is toxic to the nervous system and the kidneys.

As disturbing as all this is, the soy story may have only just begun to be told.

Soy's Underlying Link To Cancers & Infectious Diseases

The unexpected death of news anchorman, Peter Jennings, stunned millions. Appearing the picture of health, he died just months after it was announced he had lung cancer. But his was no rare, isolated instance.

Lung cancer is deadlier than breast, prostate, and colon cancers combined. In fact, it is the leading cause of all cancer deaths, advises the American Cancer Society (ACS).[1] In 1976 there were 79,000 American deaths from this disease. In 2006 more than 172,500 new cases are expected, with 163,500 such deaths anticipated. Nearly 75% of all those who develop this killer disease, die in less than two years, with no improvement of this rate in the past ten years. Too often, by the time symptoms manifest, it's too late, a physician disclosed on a morning show I heard.

Probably most people would associate lung cancer with smoking; however, a significant percentage of the victims of this deadly cancer are non-smokers. A search at SoyOnLine[2] for lung cancer, listed multiple pages of studies regarding not only lung but other soy-related cancers as well. "Why would soy and lung cancer be linked?" I wondered. A light went on.

For years my research has included periodic review of the work of Broda Barnes, MD. Dr. Barnes worked with many thousands of patients during a forty year span, with most patients suffering from previously undiagnosed hypothy- roidism. In his

---

[1] 2005 website
[2] As viewed June 2006
http://smtp.kma.co.nz/soyonlineservice/search.asp?zoom_query=soy+and+lung+cancer

very informative book, *Hypothyroidism: The Unsuspected Illness*,[1] this dedicated practitioner and scientist devoted an entire chapter to low thyroid and lung cancer. Today he would surely link these with soy. Here's why.

"Although **thyroid deficiency, as we have seen, is an important element in the development of heart attacks, hypertension, and the complications of diabetes...**," until about thirty years ago its association with cancer was not that clear-cut, explained Dr. Barnes. Then he became aware that pathologist J. G. C. Spencer of England, reported that areas of fifteen countries and four continents with low thyroid, showed higher incidences of cancer, *and especially lung cancer*. Clearly it was not coincidental that Austria, with its high incidence of hypothyroidism, also had the highest incidence of lung cancer of any country reporting malignancies.

Dr. Barnes also knew that when attempting cancer transplants in rats from one to another, rarely are such successful *"...unless the thyroid gland is removed beforehand."*

Of multiplied thousands of patients this specialist placed on thyroid therapy, *not one developed lung cancer*, and the total number developing cancer of *any* kind was approximately seventy percent less than the expected numbers in the general population. Given that some cancers are virus-related, and that "thyroid therapy increases resistance to infectious agents, including viruses responsible for colds and influenza...," the good doctor thought it worthwhile as prevention against these diseases, to check the basal temperature of every patient, and correct hypothyroidism when present.[2]

Presently, lung cancer still occurs chiefly in the elderly, the American Cancer Society tells us.[3] And great numbers of

---

[1] Barnes, B, & Galton, L, *Hypothyroidism: The Unsuspected Illness,* Harper & Row, Pub., NY, 1976-241-246

[2] Dr. Barnes' book, *Hypothyroidism: **The Unsuspected Illness,*** referred to the many physicians misdiagnosing or ignoring hypothyroidism not detected by their tests though the symptomology is present. For more information regarding the Barnes test, see that book.

[3] Netherland's Wageningen U. study shows carotenes improved lung function in srs. (*American J. Of Resp. Crit. Care & Med., 2000:161:790-795.*) Carotene defic. is linked with cancers, mac. degen., and cataracts. These nutrients work

America's aged, unable to chew meat, are turning to thyroid-suppressing soy products for protein as did the eighty-eight year old I will tell you about shortly. However, just as "couch potato" children are now experiencing diabetes II and III associated with poor diet and lack of exercise, we expect that the age of onset for some lung and other cancers, as well as infectious diseases, will also be dropping drastically.[1] Even infants are fed huge amounts of soy today. Should we also expect to see a significant increase in lung cancer in the general population as a result?

Theodore Kay of the Kyoto University of Medicine, disclosed "…thyroid enlargement in rats and humans, especially children and women, **fed with soybeans**, has been known for half a century."[2] (Enlarged thyroid signals unmet demands from the body for more of this hormone than the overworked gland is producing.)

China has 100 million women with goiters, and an epidemic of thyroid-related cretinism, according to *The New York Times*, June 4, 1996. Is this coincidental with its heavy consumption of thyroid suppressing soy products?

Soy Alert: What Took Them So Long!

The Cancer Council of New South Wales, Australia recently issued guidelines warning cancer patients and those in remission, of high soy diets and soy supplements risks.[3] They were advised to avoid these because "They can accelerate tumor growth." Research shows that high consumption of soy may also "prevent the effectiveness of conventional cancer medicines."

Soy & Breast Cancer

Estrogen dominance has been shown to be associated with a number of women's *and* men's health issues. The doctor referred

---

synergistically, are more beneficial when obtained from whole foods, not as isolates. Best source is organic eggs, followed by carrots, sweet potatoes., yams, squash, tomatoes, & green peppers.

[1] Type III diabetes is a combination of Type I juvenile and Type II adult, and is very difficult to treat.
[2] soyonlineservice.co.nz/04thyroid.htm
[3] Weaver, C, *Sunday Mail*, Adelaide, SW, Jan. 14, 2007-17

to earlier as he addressed lung cancer, also stated that this plague now strikes young women. Not surprisingly, the hostess then asked if estrogen is a factor in the new group.

Especially at risk are patients with hormone-dependent cancers, including breast and prostate cancers. Evidence suggests that women with existing or past breast cancer should be cautious in consuming large quantities of soy and soy phytoestrogen supplements, as the Australian council warned. Those in remission are "being urged to avoid high doses of soy 'as they may be more vulnerable to relapse.'"

In fact, Israeli and French governments have cautioned women who have breast cancer, or who are at risk for it, to exercise caution in consuming soy, because of the phytoestrogens (soy isoflavone) it contains, now found in myriad soy products.

The Australian council spokesman also stated that it does not support health claims on food labels suggesting that soy foods or phytoestrogens protect against cancer. Since no one knows if there is an undiscovered tumor, it would certainly seem the warning here is to all. SoyOnline Service of New Zealand laments that

> Those soy food or isoflavones supplement manufacturers that proclaim the anti-cancer properties of their products, are guilty of giving false hope to millions; but worse, they may be placing consumers at greater risk of contracting the same horrendous diseases they are trying to avoid.[1]

A Frightening Soy Event

A great-great-grandmother and her daughter, both nurses, called me about the aged mother's diet and malnourishment. The mother and daughter were working closely with the patient's medical doctor who was treating the mother chiefly for arthritis. He agreed nutritional counseling could be beneficial.

One problem was dentures that no longer fit well. Another was mail-order, high potency, vitamin isolates. Highly motivated, the client nevertheless did exceedingly well on a diet with a variety of

---

[1] soyonlineservice.co.nz/ as viewed Jan. 16, 2007

whole foods and whole-foods concentrates.[1] She was able to obtain fresh foods, even grew some on her balcony; and preferred to prepare her meals. Soon she became active again, walking a mile per day using the indoor track at the retirement center where she lived essentially independently. Later, when her doctor ordered a wheel chair for comfort and balance, she pushed it around the track.

About a year later she became very weak, to the point she was no longer ambulatory. There was nothing in the whole-foods nutritional plan that had been working so well, that should cause this. I spoke with the client and daughter, advising she be seen by her physician. He could find no reason for her acute condition. She would leave me disturbing phone messages saying she was dying, and begging for help. It was a desperate situation.

Then one day the client called and happened to mention a protein powder she had begun eating before she lost her energy, and "really liked." I asked her the source of the protein, and she responded, "Soy." She was certain it was "perfectly healthy; after all, it came from the health food store." It was "very convenient, faster than cooking and easier than chewing meat."

Upon discontinuing the product, the patient regained her strength and vitality. Today, at ninety-one years of age, she still says, "Dr. Zook saved my life!" Not really; she did. Sometimes it as simple as this: if we stop doing what prevents our wellness, and provide the body what it needs; if it is not too late, it often heals and restores itself. And sometimes even in old age.

What if this client had not thought of the soy protein powder she was taking? Would her family have prematurely lost a great influence? What do you suppose would have been shown as the cause of death on the death certificate?[2]

---

[1] By "whole foods concentrates," I mean supplements of whole foods dehydrated at low temperatures.

[2] These powders usually contain sugars that may also be problematic for glucose intolerant patients.

3 thewholesoystory.com/index.php; soyfreesolutions.com

"The Dark Side Of America's Favorite 'Health' Food"

Kaayla T. Daniel, PhD, warns us in her very informative book, *The Whole Soy Story: The Dark Side of America's Favorite Health Food,* [1]

> ...[H] **undreds** of epidemiological, clinical and laboratory studies link soy to malnutrition, infertility, digestive distress, thyroid dysfunction, birth defects, Immune System breakdown, cognitive decline, heart disease, reproductive disorders, and cancer.

Dr. Daniel likewise alerts us to "The latest ploy of the soy industry...to fan women's fears about bone loss and distract them from recent news that soy does *not* prevent heart disease, and that it worsens cardiomyopathy...and may increase breast cancer risk."[2]

Not without its thyroid problems already, China is now importing soy for unnatural fish feeding, as well as for mass production of poultry and hogs. Human consumption of soy beans, has its own problems.

Soy & Bones

A recent study from Yale-New Haven Hospital showed that "**...when soy protein is substituted for meat protein, there is an acute decline in dietary calcium bioavailability**.[3] (Remember that at least one study showed low calcium may be associated with colon cancer.) If one has accepted the misinformation that meat and even eggs cause calcium loss whereas soy protects bone, this should clear up such misapprehension and contradiction. Was it

---

[2] Daniel K, Soy and Osteoporosis: Not A Leg To Stand On, *Wise Traditions,* Vol. 7, Nr. 3, Fall 2006

[3] Kernstetter, Wall, O'Brien, Caseria, Insogna, Meat and Soy Protein Affect Calcium Homeostasis in Healthy Women; U. of Yale, CN, Cornell, *J. Nutr.* 2006;136:1890-1895.

soy or animal-based protein a great deal of the world ate successfully for many thousands of years?

American children fed soy-based milk substitutes are manifesting rickets and additional evidence of malnutrition such as used to be seen only in Third World countries.[1] One reason is that commercial soymilk may contain vitamin D_2 rather than D_3, the natural form of the vitamin/hormone. Vitamin D_2 has been linked to heart disease, allergic reactions, hyperactivity, and other conditions.

Does this sound like a safe, miracle food, and the solution to world hunger for which soy is being touted? Be sure and avail yourself of the resources mentioned at the end of this book, then decide for yourself if you haven't already.

Soy's Affect On Herpes 1

The amino acid, L-arginine, required by herpes for replication, was found by Chris Kagan, MD, Cedars of Lebanon Hospital, Los Angeles, to stimulate rapid growth of the herpes virus. R. Tankersley, MD, found that another amino acid, lysine, slows herpes' growth. Therapeutic application of L-lysine, along with reduced dietary intake of arginine, achieved excellent results without side effects, for sufferers. The critical factor was the right ratio of lysine over arginine since they compete for transport through the intestinal wall.

Chief food sources containing high and healthy lysine/arginine ratio are – you guessed it – animal-based foods beef, lamb, chicken, fish, and cheese. Foods which contain a reversed ratio, are common allergens soybeans, nuts, wheat products, and chocolate.

Lysine deficiency or excess arginine, result in concentrating difficulty, chronic tiredness, dizziness and anemia, according to University of Alabama (B'ham) researchers Ringsdorf and Cheraskin.[2]

---

[1] *Does Milk Hurt Kids?* Newsweek, May 8, 2006
[2] Chaitow L, Thorson's Guide To Amino Acids, Thorsons, London, 1991-46-47

Genetically Engineered Aberrance & Allergy

Another serious problem with soy is that except for the small amount that is organically grown, most of it is genetically engineered (GE). "Tofu, soy milk, baby formulas, soy protein shakes, protein bars, cold cereals, vegetable burgers, etc. contain GE soy *unless the label says it is organic soy* [italics supplied]."[1] Even if the soy is organic, other ingredients in the product may be GE unless they are stated to be organic.]

Eating the same food daily has been associated with food sensitivity and allergy. Soy is listed right up there with wheat, corn, and ultrapasteurized cow milk allergies.[2] Might GE soy present a "double whammy"?

Physicist Richard Wolfson, PhD, observed the UK's allergies to soy have increased a monumental fifty percent since GE soybeans came on the market.

>...[O]ne of the largest seed companies in the world created a genetically engineered soy bean a few years ago, and that soy bean was so allergic [sic], it could have killed people who were allergic to Brazil nuts. It looked exactly like every other soybean, but biochemically it was different. Luckily, they discovered it and kept it off the market. But **there is no legal requirement for the testing of these hundreds of new genetically engineered foods before they are put on the market.**[3] We do not know the long-term effects, and we need long-term testing.[4]

---

[1] Viewed Aug. 15, 2006 at consumerhealth.org/articles/display.cfm?ID=19991128220930

[2] Some people who cannot tolerate cow's milk, tolerate goat milk well. And some can tolerate raw milk who cannot tolerate ultrapasteurized milk. Some are allergic to both, after drinking an overcooked one for years.

[3] There was a recent effort to allow GE seeds to be used even in organic production; due to loud consumer outcry, FDA didn't allow it this time. To avoid GE seed, purchase organic ones.

[4] http://www.consumerhealth.org/articles/display.cfm?ID=19991128220930..

It should be understood that genetically engineering crops is more than just modification; it involves a process called transgenic manipulation, e.g., fish genes have been inserted into tomato genes. Transgenic manipulation is responsible for sheep producing human proteins in their milk, and pigs with genes for human growth hormone.[1]

And what if you are allergic to soy plus whatever else is inserted? Eating such a food might cause severe reactions in some people. Organic foods are by definition not genetically engineered.

Genetically engineered food involves far more than allergic reaction. Ronald T. Libby, PhD, University of North Florida, tells us that transgenic manipulation "…means that totally unrelated species that cannot interbreed, now can share each other's genetic composition."[2] Professor Libby continues:

> …Bioethical concerns are reflected in the term "new creationism." This refers to a subtle and dangerous attitude toward genetic engineering. It may not be safe to impose on nature a technocratic attitude toward biological systems. Rising technocracy in society values economic determinism, scientific imperialism, and **secular humanism**. This may be turning the natural world into an "industrialized wasteland" and food animals into biomachines (Fox 1990:92). The **new creationism** replaces God with humans who use the tools of molecular biology…[3]

Unborn Babies & GE Soy

A disturbing study suggests that women who eat GE soy before conception and during pregnancy, are seriously endangering their unborn babies. A leading scientist at the Russian Academy of

---

[1] Libby, RT, *The Antibiotechnology Campaign: Farmers, Food Safety Groups, and Drug Companies,* Columbia U. Press, 1998, earthscape.org/p3/libby/libby02.html
[2] *Loc. cit.*
[3] *Ibid.*

Sciences, found that more than half the offspring from rats fed GE soy flour along with other food, died in the first three weeks of life - "six times as many as born to mothers with non-modified soy or normal diets. Six times as many were also severely underweight."[1]

Genetically engineered foods and bioethics are much too complex to begin to address here; however, Dr. Libby's full article is very informative and very readable, as are many others on the Internet and elsewhere. We all *should* be concerned. Do you know what's in your non-organic foods? Check them out!

This we *will* say: now that plant genes are being *spliced* with animal genes, they are not simply genetically modified organisms (GMO), but the DNA is genetically engineered (GE). Can vegetarians be certain anymore if a vegetable is still just a vegetable? Possibly the most genetically engineered food; soy is popular with them. Most of it is not organically grown, including that sold in health food stores. If the individual ingredients are not listed as "organic," it isn't, and it is often GE.

What Of The Children, Our Next Generation?

"Vegetarian" to trendy kids means only that they don't eat meat, not that they eat even small amounts of healthy, whole foods. They are consuming chiefly simple, refined carbs; low, unhealthy fats, and soy - ubiquitous soy, GE soy.

These children are often overweight; morbid obesity is increasingly found among them. They are at risk for serious health problems, including thyroid disorder, vascular disease, and diabetes II and III.[2] Often they are "couch potatoes," get almost no exercise.

Soy is found in 60% of processed, packaged foods. Soy isoflavones (endocrine disrupters) are listed as surprise ingredients in many products where the consumer might not be expecting them, e.g. in some mayonnaise. It is also found in diet food bars, soy milk, tofu,[3] and other soy products.

---

[1] Ermakova, I, Inst of Higher Nerv Act & Neurophys, Russian Acad of Sci, Jan. 2006, Regnum News Agency (Rus)

[2] Diabetes III is a combination of types I and II, very difficult to treat.

[3] Dwyer, JT, *et al,* Tofu and soy drinks contain phytoestrogens, J Am Diet Assoc, Jul; 94(7):739-43.

It may promote precocious puberty (premature sexual development) in little girls; while delaying puberty and leading to feminization in boys due to isoflavones' inhibition of an enzyme that is vital in testosterone development.[1] One physician, Chris Meletis, ND, describes it thus:

> A sad fact is that young boys are now suffering gynemastia, a condition that causes them to develop breasts as though they were young girls. This condition in males used to be seen in older men, and those that drank alcohol to excess....These days, boys suffer not only the self-esteem issues common to boys their ages, but their bodies manifest a consequence of estrogen [soy phytoestrogen] that destroys more than just their natural pride - it increases risk for cancer, and much more.[2]

It is disturbing to do an on-line search and view the numbers of websites dealing with these concerns of many young men and boys. Men are now undergoing chest reductions.

It appears these issues may have even more to do with the mother's prenatal diet with soy, and fixation of gender in utero, ending in confusion for the child.[3] What of the combination of the prenatal and after-birth soy diets of some infants given soy milk and cereal?

An incredible number of boy babies are now born with what was once a rare condition known as hypospadias. This tragic deformity of the penis in which the opening lies somewhere in the underside of the penile shaft instead of at the end of it, includes a shortening of the penis as well – as much as 2.6 inches in severe cases.[4]

---

[1] Biochem. Biophys. Res. Commun. 195 Oct. 24:215, 3, 1137-44
[2] Email 3/07
[3] Homosexual young males are 14 times more likely to attempt suicide during their youth. They amounted to 63% of suicide attempts in a Calgary study. fsw.ucalgary.ca/ramsay/homosexuality-suicide/05-quebec-suicide-paper.htm
[4] Baskin, L, Hypospadias and Genital Development, Advances in Experimental Biology and Medicine," Vol. 545., Kluwer Academic/Plenum Publishers, NY, 2004

Overall, the malformity is associated with homosexuality; one small study showed that 7.6 percent of the control (healthy) subjects were exclusively homosexual compared with 20.3 percent of those with hypospadias (plus another 15.5 percent who were bisexual).[1]

In the UK, vegetarian mothers, likely drinking soy milk as 40% of Brits do, are giving birth to hypospadias babies in one of 25 births, five times the usual risk.[2] The 1999 Australia/New Zealand Food Authority (ANZFA), now Food Standards/ Australia/NZ, wrote an Assessment of the Potential Risk To Infants Associated with Exposure To Soy-based Infant Formulas. One paragraph of the 50 page document reads as follows:

> While it is clear that phyto**estrogens** pose a potential hazard to the consumer of soy foods, they are also suggested to have benefits. The hazard consists of the potential changes in hormone levels in adults and infants, and includes effects arising from estrogen agonism, anti-estrogenic activity, reduction in thyroid function, and alteration of sex-specific patterns of early development.[3]

Soy & Children's Leukemia

Scientific evidence now links phytoestrogen of soy products with a shocking increase in the incidence of leukemia in children. The latest figures show an alarming 27% in one year in America.[4]

Deadly Silence

Why is all this scandalous, scientific evidence not big news, and why are these products with such grave and frightening

---

[1] Rutz J, The Trouble With Soy, Part 5, *World Net Daily*, Jan. 9, 2007 wnd.com/news/article.asp?ARTICLE_ID=53675
[2] North, K, Golding, J, A maternal diet in pregnancy is associated with hypospadias. BJU Int, 2000:35, 107-13
[3] Tomaska, L, et al, Assessment of the Potential Risk to Infants Associated With Exposure to Soy-Based Infant Formulas, Mar. 1999, ANZFA doc., Sec. 6 p. 29
[4] Rutz, J, *Soy Is Making Kids "Gay,"* WorldNetDaily, Dec. 12, 2006

potential, not taken off the market? In an experiment, after just two weeks of drinking eight ounces of soy milk daily ("70 mg. of soy isoflavones per serving"), my temperature dropped a full degree; my metabolism slowed significantly – both pointing to an affected thyroid. Soy savvy Valerie and Richard James, wrote:

> The effects of soy on our parrots' thyroids and reproduction, extended at least three generations in the few that retained some degree of fertility. That's what really worried us for the implications for kids fed soy formulas...
>
> The Old Testament warning that the sins of the fathers could extend unto the fourth generation, occurred to us...As a learned professor said..., "It was not too disastrous when it was confined to a family or a village, but this industry has turned it into a world-wide problem."[1]

In May 2007, a six week old Georgia infant died after being fed a diet of soy milk, apple juice, and breast milk from a vegan mother presumably drinking soy milk before, during the pregnancy, and while nursing.[2] I could find no mention of soy isoflavones on the label of a recent soy "milk" container, though there was a warning that it is not to be used as infant formula. that very likely contained soy isoflavones (endocrine disrupters suppressing the thyroid) and perhaps was GE. The parents of the three and one-half pound emaciated infant, received life sentences.

What will be the state of the offspring of even this generation raised on environmental estrogens, low protein/low fat non-foods, without phytonutrients from fruits and vegetables – assuming most are capable of procreation. (Since the devitalization and denaturing of the American diet and the onset of the Standard American Diet (SAD) beginning in the 1920's, studies show infertility has risen from ten to a tragic forty percent in the US. Later we will see this barrenness duplicated in a study of forty generations of cats

---

[1] Personal communication, Jan. 2007
[2] Macklin W, Vegan Parents Get Life In Prison For Death Of Son, AHN, alheadlinenews.com/articles/7007293107

suffering increasing malnutrition as a result of not being fed according to God's plan for eating for them.)

Babe's Powerful Influence

It is important to know why our Christian youth are increasingly becoming vegetarian, even radical vegans. Some of those reasons may surprise you.

A friend in Australia related how her young daughter was strongly influenced against eating meat as a result of viewing the American movie, *Babe*. We almost never go to movies; however, I too viewed this one, thought it a very enjoyable fairy tale. Yet children often don't differentiate between make-believe and reality. Secular humanism taught by public schools, declares that humans are only more highly evolved animals – thus logic tells children that *eating meat is cannibalism*.

They don't want animals killed for human food even though they may wear leather garments. In the food chain, animals eat one another and that is acceptable to vegetarians, because those animals couldn't survive if they didn't.

Movies are not the only strong influence toward vegetarianism in our children's lives today. School teachers and other authority figures, peers, and TV are some other strong influences.

Often family TV programs show people kissing animals' mouths, and animals passionately licking the faces of their owners.[1] Children constantly hear pet owners tell their pets, "Come to Mommy;" or "Go to Daddy." "Animals are family too;" or "Animals are people too," children also hear often. Pets have human names, sleep with their owners (how much longer will we be called "owners" of our pets?), and in general are treated as humans as much as possible. Christmas gifts for dogs of perfume and purses were pitched in 2006. Today's children's thinking, including Christian children's thinking, is skewed in this regard, for good reason.

---

[1] Have they never seen the same animals licking their own anuses with parasite ova (e.g. tapeworms) and filth of wherever they've been?

The Root Of Kids' Confusion

Our kids are taught by numerous sources, that as evolved animals, humans are not superior to them; and that all living things are plant and animal, not plant, animal, and human beings as Genesis 1 declares. Jesus Christ taught that humans are superior to animals.[1] No wonder kids are confused! Here is an example of such. Alison Green's website states:

> ...[V]egetarianism means no red meat, poultry, or fish - **nobody with a face**...Especially if someone is a vegetarian for ethical reasons, don't assume they won't object to "just a little" meat in their meal. **Would you accept "just a bit" of your cat, or "just a little" of Uncle Jim in your soup?**[2]

This confusion is the inevitable consequence of non-acceptance of humans as a separate, sole classification, the only creature made in God's image. It demonstrates an inability to differentiate between humans and animals, including those animals God created to be eaten by man. (Man was not created to be eaten by any creature.)

Ms. Green, who became a vegan because of her values, says she eats spaghetti, hummus, sorbet, soup, salads, burritos, gingerbread, lentil chili, lasagna, tofu kabobs, waffles, vegetable burgers, artichokes, tacos, bagels, rice, and other foods.[3] There is a surprising lack of vegetables in Green's diet considering she is a **veg**etarian. However, the lack of protein and fats in a very high carb diet, is typical of this diet, also chiefly accounting for America's burgeoning bellies and a 60% overweight population.

Says a New Age former vegan concerned that they are "in the dark:"

> If you don't care about your own health, or if you're willing to sacrifice your own health because of the ethical considerations for the animal world, then I don't have any problems with that. If a person knows that they're going to

---

[1] Matt. 10:31
[2] Available at http://www.eatveg.com/harmony.htm on Mar. 25, 2006
[3] Green A, Living in Harmony with Vegetarians, *The Washington Post*, Aug. 25, 1995

have an increased chance of dying prematurely, and having different health problems, but are choosing that path **knowingly**, because of their love for the animal world, well then that's fine...[1]

This Essene pastor's concern is that most vegans *do not know* – at least for some time - that they are sacrificing their health and possibly their lives, for animals. Worse, he says, they are being lied to by hypocritical leaders. We will address this hypocrisy, and his very brave stand, later in this book.

Death Is Essential For Life

Few children today have farm roots and understand the cycles of life. They are not aware that death is part of life, is necessary in fact to produce life. Only one sperm survives each pregnancy; all the countless others die. Jesus said a kernel of grain must fall into the ground and die in order to bring forth many more kernels to feed many. Seed corn is saved for this purpose, and vegans do not object to a seed sacrificed to give life for more grain to feed humans.

The fact is that since time began, life has always required death. Prairie grass thrived on dead and composted plants, and fed the buffalo herds, that in turn died to feed the American Indians, the pioneers and settlers. There can be no life without death.[2] Vegetarians seem to pretend this is not so, and ignore much else.

Did God Forget Something?

Today's inadequate vegetarian diet is "propped up" in particular with soy, an inferior source of protein. Neither do beans and grains have the important nutrients of flesh-foods; they are not a long term substitute for meat, fish and fowl.

If the Creator intended for mankind to be vegetarian, one

---

[1] Nazariah, New Age Essene Church of Christ, rawfoodinfo.com/hotline/Sept04Part3_hotline.html, Nov. 2006

[2] The death of the Lord Jesus Christ is the greatest example of one death producing life for countless others.

would think He would have provided a variety of non-flesh foods with quality, complete proteins in one food, found round the world. Further, Scripture would demonstrate that from Genesis to Revelation. Instead, we have a strong warning to the contrary to which we have devoted a great deal of this book. More later.

Before going on, let's be clear that God's Word plainly declares that abstaining from meat that He created to be eaten, will be powerfully promoted in the end time. Soy has replaced meats for many, including many Christians unfortunately, based upon the wisdom of man.

Yet in spite of what millions have heard from countless sources, soy beans appear to be similar to other legumes in that they are deficient in sulfur-containing amino acids methionine and cystine (provided by eggs).

Besides the amino acid arginine/lysine ratio, the denaturing of amino acids by processing, may present an additional issue with soy protein as a satisfactory substitute for complete protein.[1]

Soy industry products are fast reaching a great percentage of the globe. Did God intend this ubiquitous substance to meet world protein needs in these last days? If so, why is it not once mentioned in the Bible?

As we have seen, and will further develop, that great book of wisdom for the ages, *does* tell us what that source is to be.

This chapter is dedicated to the memory of Valerie James who valiantly and persistently fought against soy foods including its use in infant formula. Valerie passed away February 23, 2008, but her valiant work will continue for our benefit and for the generations to come…

---

[1] Soy OnLine Service, *Myths & Truths About Soy*, soyonlineservice.co.nz/03soymyths.htm, Dec. 2006

8

Vegetarianism –
Is It Scientifically Sound?

Works Versus Grace

The first murder had to do with vegetable versus animal.[1] Cain's vegetable sacrifice, representing sinful man's effort (works) to earn his salvation and atone for his sin, was unacceptable to Jehovah. Abel's lamb was approved; for "…without the shedding of blood, there is no remission of sin," Hebrews 9:22 teaches us. Vegetarianism is still unacceptable to God.

An Overview

"Do you not therefore err, because you know not the Scriptures, neither the power of God?" Jesus responded to those drawing conclusions with incomplete knowledge of His Word.[2] And that is the chief issue today regarding God's dietary plan after the Fall.

This chapter deals with vegetarianism in the broad sense, as a diet that does not include flesh foods but may include dairy (lacto vegetarianism) and/or eggs (ova vegetarianism).[3] Vegetarianism "comes in many flavors;" but this is how most understand a vegetarian diet. It does not require killing an animal, repugnant to

---

[1] Gen. 4
[2] Mark 12:24
[3] Pescatarians eat fish, and thus are not true vegetarians. Since fish "have a face," pescatarian logic is hard to explain.

this group.[1] Most of the dietary intake is carbohydrate, with multiple, serious inadequacies of vital nutrients, as we shall reveal shortly.

Veganism, the subject of the next chapter, includes those who don't consume any animal-resource foods. Vegans may be divided into 2 groups: those who eat cooked and raw foods; and those who eat all foods raw. All vegans are vegetarians, but not all vegetarians are vegans. Chapter Eight addresses this extreme form of vegetarianism. This rapidly growing group includes multiplied millions of Americans. It includes New Agers, teens, and others; as well as a significant number of Christians, contrary to the Word of God and sound nutrition science. All of these sub-groups, are rapidly increasing.

Vegetarianism & Sex Hormones

What the Puerto Ricans call *chispa de la vita*, the spark of life, often seems lacking in vegetarians. Often they have "blah," difficult, or weak personalities. The voice of one nationally-known, vegetarian physician has no force; his wife is appears emaciated, one can hardly hear her speak for lack of vitality.

Visiting a vegetarian medical doctor's message board was enlightening. There were more than 50 complaints from husbands whose vegetarian wives had no libido. Young vegetarian males reported low testosterone, suffering from erectile dysfunction (EF), and low sperm count. Testosterone makes a man a man.

Vegetarian diets are also often low-fat diets. Fats are essential for the body's production of steroid hormones. Combine this deficiency with phytoestrogen from soy products, and we have confused, effeminate young men thinking themselves to be homosexual. In fact, many may be suffering from malnutrition, especially with a fat-deficient diet leading to low sex hormone levels; and estrogen dominance from high soy isoflavones intake.

CAUTION: It can be helpful to work with a qualified practitioner when attempting to change your diet. Readers should be aware that anyone can – and they *do* – call themselves "nutritionists." Some may be multilevel marketing distributors or

---

[1] We will address the hypocrisy of this further on.

medical doctors, with little or no formal education in nutrition.[1] Dieticians may have little training in whole foods nutrition and supplementation. Comparatively few practitioners may use whole foods concentrates with their clients and patients.[2]

If such counseling is needed, try to work with at least a certified nutritionist trained in fresh, whole foods such as you will be learning here and in the forthcoming book about whole foods. Such practitioners are "scarce as hens' teeth." Pray for God's provision for that which you need to improve your health to His glory and use. Many naturopaths and chiropractors have some training or are self-taught in nutrition though usually not in whole foods and whole foods concentrates. These *Eatin' After* Eden books can provide a strong foundation supporting increased levels of wellness as well.

The Best Vegetarian Diets Aren't Enough

Vegetarian diets vary in their deficiencies, largely depending upon how much animal food they include or lack. Lacto-ovo vegetarians (including dairy and eggs), may suffer least. Even so, they are not consuming God-ordained, optimum nutrition. Only flesh foods, with their exceptionally high quality protein, provide the body with the ideal amino acids ratio.

Though most people think of meat as any flesh food, actually only red meat is "meat," other animal foods are poultry, (chicken, turkey, et al), and fish. The King James Bible, is correct in its referring to all such foods as flesh foods. However, in this book we may sometimes refer to any flesh food as "meat" as it is called today, for the sake of understanding.

Red meats (e.g., beef, lamb, wild game) have nutrients not found in poultry and fish, some perhaps yet unknown. We have previously discussed CLA that is found only in red meat and milk fat. I know of a case where one suffers chronic headaches and neck pain unless red meat is consumed regularly. Nothing else takes care of it. Another case has to do with severe panic attacks and

---

[1] Medical students may have one semester of "basic nutrition," but usually not.
[2] "Whole foods concentrates" refers here to supplements made entirely of whole foods as grown in (organic) soil.

depression that is relieved only by the person's eating red meat. The same nutrients from other sources are ineffective for her.

Ideally, one would consume a variety of animal flesh as listed in Leviticus 11 and Deuteronomy 14. We need all three groups: meats, poultry, and fish. However, for some people it is best to eat only one type meat each day, alternating at least every four days if one suffers food allergies, or to prevent them.

We enjoy non-meat meals when we eat other complete protein, e.g. eggs, cheese, cottage cheese, and complementary proteins. Smoothies with whey or goat milk protein powder from the health food store are also occasional options when cooking is not convenient or desired. However, not even these protein powders provide other nutrients found in flesh foods.

Vegetarian Diets' Missing Nutrients

Many people believe that *only* vitamin B_{12} is missing from vegan diets. And no wonder when authoritarian, seemingly credible and well known leaders teach this strongly. One such medical doctor writes, "B-12 is the only legitimate criticism of a healthy vegan diet." In fact, he went on to state dogmatically, "There are no other nutritional deficiencies caused by a vegan diet of whole plant foods – in other words, **there is no chance** of calcium, amino acid [sic], protein, vitamin D, essential fatty acid, zinc, or iron deficiency – except B12 deficiency."[1] This doctor, most of whose colleagues would not agree with him, confuses the Standard American Diet (SAD), "a typical B-12-sufficient diet," with eating meat. Because one eats meat and a "B-12 sufficient diet," certainly does not mean they consume the "Western diet," he also speaks about. Of course we do not consume or recommend the typical Western diet (the SAD)!

Beginning with vitamin B_{12}, the following list includes multiple nutrients commonly missing from vegetarian diets. Some of the chief benefits of the missing nutrients are also included here in order that you might understand that a diet deficient in these

---

[1] McDougall, J, *Back to the Garden,* Summer 2003, Iss. Nr. 24, "from the McDougall Newsletter," as published by George H. Malkmus & Hallelujah Acres.

nutrients, may present a serious health risk. In the next chapter we will discuss veganism in particular, and its additional deficiencies.

Vitamin B$_{12}$: Another post-Eden priority, this nutrient is safe even at mega doses. The term "B$_{12}$" actually represents a family of compounds containing the mineral cobalt. Hence "*cobalamin*"(Cbl) is used when referring to compounds with B$_{12}$ activity. It is a critically important nutrient found only in animal products since the Fall. Excellent sources are liver, eggs, canned herring, beef, milk, and cheese.

Medical schools and dieticians teach that vitamin B$_{12}$ is found naturally in *lean* red meat, *skinless* chicken, and *skim* (low fat) milk you will recognize from Chapter Three and the PD. Our grass-fed, red meat was naturally lean until the steers were about 18 months of age; whereas what is usually meant by "lean red meat" is fatty meat with the outer layers of fat trimmed. What they've done to the Creator's whole foods - in the pasture and the kitchen - is not nutrition but *mal*nutrition in my opinion!

Many conditions are prevented by this nutrient. It is vital for cellular "operation," for the formation of red blood cells and proteins, and normal functioning of the central nervous system. It is involved in energy release from the macronutrients as well. Vegetarians as well as non-vegetarians who avoid healthy sources of this vitamin, or those who suffer malfunctioning stomachs, intestines and pancreas, may be commonly deficient in the essential nutrient.

Sadly, we commonly see vitamin B$_{12}$ deficiency in seniors for whom it is associated with neurological disorders. This is not due to aging, *per se,* but poor diets and inadequate digestion and absorption, all of which can often and easily be improved by supplementation administered by a qualified health care practitioner.

Vitamin B$_{12}$ deficiency can also lead to a deficiency of the active form of folate, another B vitamin. Folate is important *before* and during the first weeks of pregnancy to reduce the risk of neural tube defects, affecting the brain and spinal cord of the unborn baby.[1] Normal formation and regeneration of red blood cells requires folate. It is important for reducing blood homocysteine levels, and for protein metabolism. It has been shown to prevent osteoporosis-related fractures and dementias, including the dreaded Alzheimer's disease.[2] If you are irritable, suffer gingivitis, memory loss, or confusion; fatigue - mental and muscle - even insomnia, you may need more folate.

Folate deficiency is seen when there is a lack of God-ordained, animal based and green foods as commanded in Genesis 9:3.[3] Chicken and calf livers provide highest sources. Dark green, leafy vegetables are a lesser but good source.

A deficiency of vitamin B_{12} is associated with megaloblastic anemia,[4] bone spurs, bursitis, canker sores, poor fingernails, weakness and excessive fatigue, rosacea, sciatica, senility, and shingles. Some other signs are a variety of psychiatric disorders, including depression, disorientation, mood disturbance, memory loss, irritability, and dementia. Paresthesia (numbness and tingling in the hands and legs) may be present as well. Or the deficiency may manifest with an inability to maintain balance while walking. Even irregular menstrual cycles may result from this deficiency. Clearly, rejecting God's plan for eating can result in serious conditions.

This critical nutrient is essential for mental and lower extremity proper development of babies. Vegans' babies have died due to this lack.[5] Children need it for growth and appetite. Mental concentration is also associated with this vitamin. It is important

---

[1] By the time a woman defic. in this vit. knows she is pg., damage may have already been done to her unborn child.

[2] *The World's Healthiest Foods*, as viewed 12/3/06.
whfoods.com/genpage.php?tname=nutrient&dbid=63

[3] Folic acid is very heat sensitive. Try to eat your dark, green leafy vegetables raw or lightly steamed.

[4] For many years it was believed that anemia was the first sign of B_{12} deficiency. More recently we are seeing neurological damage linked to this deficiency, where anemia is not present.

[5] Unless supplementing this, vegan mothers' milk does not contain this vitamin critical for nursing infants. See also
http://www.second-opinions.co.uk/child_abuse.html, and
http://chetday.com/hallelujah-diet-baby.htm

for energy, and another one of many nutrients good bones require, especially in older people.[1]

Vegans may depend upon vitamin B_{12} being produced by certain intestinal bacteria. If it is, it is not reliably utilized since vitamin B_{12} requires binding with intrinsic factor for proper absorption in the ileum. Very few vitamin B_{12} supplements include intrinsic factor, a protein produced by stomach lining glands.

Besides digesting protein, stomach acid also releases vitamin B_{12} from food. Thus vitamin B_{12} deficiency may be associated with low hydrochloric acid. (An acquaintance related her experience with "heart burn" as a result of food fermenting in her stomach from lack of adequate hydrochloric acid. She said she didn't wish to purchase a digestive enzyme formula costing $24.95 [her greater priority was a new puppy costing $300], whereupon she then was told she might instead invest in a teaspoon of raw apple cider vinegar in a glass of water with meals. Unfortunately she decided to skip the water, took the vinegar straight, and burned her esophagus.)

Healthy nervous systems and nerve sheaths require B_{12}. Like others of the B vitamin complex, it helps with proper utilization of protein, carbohydrates and fats.

Due to its being "recycled" in the blood, a vitamin B_{12} deficiency may not be evident for years. Further, if the diet is low in vitamin B_{12} and high in folic acid as found in vegetarian diets, a B_{12} deficiency is often hidden. The founder and leader of one such diet group, had been a vegan for years before he announced his B_{12} deficiency and advised his followers to supplement this vitamin.

Some people are unable to digest and absorb vitamin B_{12} even in animal-based food.[2] Sublingual supplementation may help though it may not be well absorbed and is limited in utilization. Supplementation in its finest form cannot begin to duplicate the intricate array of nutrients contained in animal-based foods as designed and prescribed by the Creator Himself.

Vitamin B_{12} and folate function interdependently to form red blood cells, and produce thymidine, an essential building block of

---

[1] Green & Kinsella, *Current concepts in the diagnosis of cobalamin deficiency*, *Neurology*, Aug. 1995, 45, 1435-1440

[2] When stomach acid or the intrinsic factor are low.

DNA. It is required for preservation and transfer of genetic information.

For many years, raw cow's liver was used successfully to cure conditions associated with vitamin B_{12} deficiencies, including neurological damage and pernicious anemia.

If you are considering being tested for B_{12} deficiency, you may wish to use the urine test. Green and Kinsella discovered that serum B_{12}, the most widely used screening test for this deficiency, is not reliable. It "...lacks both sensitivity and specificity for diagnosis of this deficiency owing to numerous technical and interpretive problems."[1] Urine may produce more reliable test results, though there are better howbeit more complicated ones.[2] You may wish to order a copy of the Green/Kinsell study abstract from your local library for your physician and discuss it with him/her.

NOTE: A number of products are advertised as excellent vitamin B_{12} sources when they are not. Fermented soy (tempeh and miso), shiitake mushrooms, and algae products, have little if any active vitamin B_{12}. Their analogs of this critical vitamin are not active, they may even prevent absorption of the real nutrient.

We have seen that from a vegan diet it is impossible to get quality protein that is easily digested and contains vitamin B_{12}. The first humans may have produced it in adequate amounts before the Fall, or had other resources. But since the Fall, animal products are the only reliable food sources. This alone is strong reason to believe that *man did not continue a vegan diet after Eden*. This critical nutrient and other important ones listed here, cannot be obtained from plant foods, at least today. Yet this vitamin and quality protein are not the only important nutrients lacking in many vegetarian diets. Here are some others.

Vitamin A: Vegetarians consider beta-carotene (β–carotene) to be vitamin A. Actually beta-carotene is a provitamin and precursor that must be converted to vitamin A; it is *not* vitamin A (retinol).[3]

---

[1] Neurology, Aug. 1995
[2] *Ibid.*
[3] Regarding toxic amounts of real vit. A, see westonaprice.org/modernfood/codliver-manufacture.html

Six units of the provitamin are required for one unit of vitamin A, however, just taking six times the number of units of vitamin A you desire, does not mean that you will get adequate vitamin A. It's not nearly that simple; nor will consuming gallons of carrot juice alone provide vitamin A.

Bile salts in the intestine are necessary for this conversion and absorption, requiring fat to be eaten with the beta-carotene in order to stimulate the secretion of bile from the gallbladder. Yet many Americans may suffer from gallbladder issues, at least in part due to low-fat diets. Additionally, increasing numbers are dealing with thyroid and diabetes problems that may inhibit the conversion. Neither are infants' intestines capable of producing vitamin A from beta-carotene.[1]

True, this carotene is a valuable nutrient, however, if you take beta-carotene as an isolated antioxidant, how do you know how much to take? How much carrot juice should you drink? The many types of antioxidants perform different functions. Supplement advertising doesn't tell us that they're not all good. Antioxidants can and do deactivate free radicals *in vitro* (test tube), but in our bodies they may have the opposite effect, sometimes acting as pro-oxidants instead, forming oxidized by-products, especially if adequate amounts of vitamins C and E are absent, as shown by two β–carotene studies.[2]

Real vitamin A is essential for skin, eyes, lung development, calcium absorption and bone formation; reproduction, immunity, and a great deal more. It is preformed and fat soluble, requiring fat for efficient absorption. This extremely important nutrient is found only in animal foods, especially cod liver oil, liver, egg yolks, butter, cream, and cheese from grass-fed cows. Oswald A. Roels, PhD, Associate Professor of Nutrition at Columbia University, discovered an interdependence between dietary protein and vitamin A: that "...[V]itamin A is vital to proper absorption and use of protein."[3]

---

[1] Jennings, I, *Vitamins in Endocrine Metabolism,* Chas. Thomas, London, 1970-39-57
[2] CARET Study 1996; Finnish study 1994, *Wellness Guide To Dietary Supplements,* UC Berkley Wellness Letter, March 2000
[3] *New York State Journal of Medicine,* Jan. 15, 1964, as reported in *The Complete Book of Vitamins,* Rodale, JI, Rodale Books, 1975-60-61

When 500 Indonesian children suffering from protein deficiency kwashiorkor, were given vitamin A along with the same amount of protein previously fed, there was "far more increase in height and weight." On the other hand, Dr. Roels found that a protein deficiency "made it more difficult to absorb and utilize vitamin A, so that the two nutrients were shown to work far better together for the promotion and maintenance of health that neither could do separately." Do you suppose the Creator knew this when He added vitamin A to liver, egg yolks, and cheese with their quality protein?

Vitamin D_3: Chiefly known for calcium absorption and bone metabolism, this vitamin/hormone is required for literally thousands of biochemical processes. Made from that long "four letter word," cholesterol, it may be obtained from diet, or from sunlight acting upon the skin - *if* there is adequate cholesterol under the skin and all else is physiologically fit for the job. It is found chiefly in animal-based foods cod liver oil, egg yolks, fatty fish, butter,[1] and milk.

Not surprisingly, vegan/vegetarian diets are quite deficient in vitamin D_3. In fact, "Food, excluding cod liver oil, as a primary source of this nutrient, is difficult to impossible" to find, advises vitamin D expert Kristin Sullivan, CN.[2] Cod liver oil, with its vitamins A, D, and F all three, is very important for moving calcium from the intestine to where it is needed.

The safety of vitamin D_2, known as ergocalciferol, (a synthetic vitamin not to be confused with naturally occurring D_3) has been questioned and found wanting by more than a few. In fact, the "synthetic vitamin D2, added to milk, actually has the opposite effect of naturally occurring vitamin D complex, causing decalcification of the hard tissues and calcification of the soft tissues, including the soft tissues of the arteries."[3]

---

[1] Even pasteurized butter may include all the very valuable, fat soluble vitamins – A, D, E, & K.

[2] Sullivan, K, *The Miracle of Vitamin D,* Weston A. Price Foundation, as viewed June 26, 2006 at
http://www.westonaprice.org/basicnutrition/vitamindmiracle.html

[3] Buist RA. Vit Tox, *Side Effects and Contdications*. Int Clncl Nutr Review 4(4), 159-171, 1984

In recent years many exciting studies have been undertaken with vitamin D_3 suggesting that the RDA of 400 IU/day and even the Food and Nutrition Board's previously defined Upper Limit (UL) of 2,000 IU/day may be perilously low.

Research shows there are vitamin D receptors not only in the gut and bone, but especially in the brain, breast, lymphocytes, and prostate. Later research suggests "higher vitamin D levels provide protection from diabetes mellitus, osteoporosis, osteoarthritis, hypertension, cardiovascular disease, metabolic syndrome, depression, several autoimmune diseases, and cancers of the breast, prostate and colon..."[1]

Increasingly, research has pointed to this vitamin deficiency in the presence of bone and muscle pain, and severe muscle weakness; thus patients may be offered preventative and therapeutic applications of this nutrient as never before. [2]

A Portland, Oregon veteran's hospital study "...indicated that high vitamin D is more strongly linked to colon health than high calcium use, which previous studies have linked to intestinal health." People consuming higher amounts of this vitamin had "fewer serious colon polyps than others," a common concern.[3] *If a nutrient will prevent a disease, might not a deficiency of same, lead to that condition?*

According to the William B. Grant analysis, breast cancer risk could be cut fifty percent with sufficient vitamin D levels. Prevention of prostate cancer with this vitamin/hormone, also looks promising in ongoing studies.

Now consider this: all your life you have been told that you are getting plenty of this vitamin from the sun and the food industry. Yet a Harvard Medical School study showed that 57% of the hospital patients involved in the study were deficient in vitamin D and 22% were *severely* deficient.[4] Professor Paresh Dadonda, MD, also "...found severe deficiency of the vitamin in a cohort of

---

[1] Vasquez, Manso, & Cannell, *The Clncl Ime Of Vit D (Cholecalciferol): A Paradigm Shift With Impl For All HealthCare Providers*, Integ Med, Vol. 3, Nr. 5, Oct./Nov. 2004-44

[2] Dadona P, Dept. of Med, SUNY, Buffalo, buffalo.edu/news/fast-execute.cgi/expert-page.html?expert=550012

[3] Dworkin, A, Vitamin D linked to colon health, *The Oregonian*, Dec. 11, 2003

[4] New Eng. Jnl. of Med. (NEJM) 98; 338(12): 777-783

Kashmiri women, related to wearing of heavy clothing and the burkah."[1]

A Swedish study reported in February of 2006, showed that people over 65 years of age, have weak lower muscles that cause falls (leading to broken hips and death). High vitamin D intake reduced the number of falls by 50% during the three year study.[2]

"If you're taking estrogen in an effort to treat osteoporosis, it may be the equivalent of burning down the barn to get rid of the mice," warns Timothy Long, ND, an internationally recognized naturopathic physician. "What most women aren't told is that *vitamin D has the same positive effect on bone mass as estrogen – without the associated cancer risk.*"[3] Is that amazing or what! Not really, for thousands of years women thrived on animal-based foods and sunshine. They had no breast cancer. They were active outdoors a great deal more than many women today.

If you are a vegan eating a low-fat diet, fearing sunshine, and you get only 400 IU of vitamin D from your supplements, what do you think may be your level of adequacy of this another extremely important nutrient?[4] If you suffer fat maldigestion, or if you have had your gallbladder removed, a before-meals bile supplement may be suggested for you by a qualified natural physician.

Mothers can start infants off right with prenatal cod liver oil.[5] A recent Canadian study shows that when pregnant women take this nutrient, it helps prevent low birth weight.

Calcium: "Calcium is essential for every vital bodily function. It plays an important role in utilization of vitamins. Many diseases and conditions are said to be directly or indirectly related to calcium deficiency."[6] Other minerals must be in right ratio to calcium, and vice versa. You may have heard the saying, "If mama

---

[1] Dadona P, *Ibid.*
[2] Feb. 3, 2006, CBS News.
[3] Long, T, The Epidemic of Vitamin D Deficiencies, *The Pathlighter* IACVF, Oct. 1998
[4] For further info regarding the myth that sunshine is all you need for vit. D, see also WAPF's westonaprice.org/mythstruths/mtvegetarianism.html#3
[5] For detailed info about cod liver oil's processing and potency, see westonaprice.org/modernfood/codliver-manufacture.html
[6] Zook, S, *NW Senior News*, Nov. 2004

ain't happy, ain't nobody happy." It's like that with calcium; if it's not balanced with other nutrients required for its utilization, it seems nothing else is. There can be no "mama" without a family of other nutrients to support it. I have provided that list as Exhibit A at the end of this chapter.

Taurine: This is the most concentrated amino acid in the heart muscle; and it is required for all muscles. It is not found in vegetable protein, only in animal-based foods. Taurine is a "...remarkable accessory food factor..." that may be synthesized in the body; however, nutrition scientist Jeffrey Bland, PhD, advises that "...vegetarians on a diet containing imbalanced protein intake...may have difficulty manufacturing taurine..." in their bodies.[1]

The hormone estradiol depresses the formation of taurine in the liver, as may phytoestrogens of soy isoflavones. Additional estradiol in the form of medication increases this inhibition.[2]

Taurine is also required by the entire central nervous system. It acts as a calming neurotransmitter for the brain. White blood cells require this almost-essential amino acid, as does bile for detoxification and fat digestion. It is critical for absorption of fat soluble vitamins A, D, E and K, as well as control of blood fats (serum cholesterol). It helps prevent retinal degeneration as well. Taurine (from the Latin *bos taurus,* bovine) is particularly important for its sulfur for detoxification of today's myriad synthetic chemicals and toxic metals in our environment. Sulfur deficiency is associated with poor muscle tone, arthritis, skin issues, nervous system weakness, and low libido.[3]

Taurine helps metabolize fat from the animal-based foods in which it is found. Recall that eggs are a chief source of sulfur and not surprisingly, this critical amino acid is as well. Again, it is not found in vegetable protein.

Threonine: This EAA is supportive of cardiovascular, central nervous and immune systems (it aids in the production of

---

[1] Chaitow, L, Thorsons, *Thorson's Guide To Amino Acids*, London, 1991-68
[2] Chaitow, 69
[3] *Essential Oils Desk Reference,* Essential Science Pub., 2000-366

antibodies). It is found in high concentrations in the heart and skeletal muscles. An important constituent of collagen, elastin, bone, and enamel protein, its richest sources include meats, poultry, dairy foods, and eggs. Dear reader, are you beginning to see why the Creator gave us animal-based foods?

Threonine also helps prevent the fatty liver associated with low protein diets.[1] Considered an essential for good mental health, a deficiency may be associated with irritabilty and personality disorders, and generally difficult or cantankerous patients, according to nutrition researcher, W. M. Ringsdorf, DMD, at the University of Alabama (Birmingham).[2] (As an undergrad student and patient, I worked with Dr. Ringsdorf at the beginning of my very long and complicated journey for health.)

Further, inadequate threonine may lead to indigestion, malabsorption and malnourishment.[3] Nutrients are better absorbed when this EAA is in the diet.

This is another very important EAA often found lacking in vegan diets, along with lysine. Missing from most grains, it can only be obtained with great effort in vegan diets. It requires combining right amounts of properly prepared and soaked legumes which *do* contain threonine plus lysine, in right amounts of (pre-soaked) grain, if vegans are to get complete protein.[4] Not only must the beans and grains be in right ratios, they must be cooked at low temperatures else this critical amino acid is destroyed. How many vegans know this, much less do it?

Zinc: This is a critical component of numerous vital enzymes. It is important for a healthy immune system, wound healing, sense of taste and smell, and for DNA synthesis. This mineral also supports normal growth and development during pregnancy, childhood, and into adolescence.

Signs and symptoms of a deficiency of this mineral include anorexia, growth retardation, delayed sexual maturation,

---

[1] Borrmann, W., *Comprehensive Answers to Nutrition,* New Horizon, Chicago, 1979
[2] Cheraskin & Ringsdorf, *Psychodietetics,* Bantam, 1976
[3] Chaitow, *Op cit.*, p. 176
[4] Davis, A., *Let's Eat Right to Keep Fit,* George Allen & Unwin, London, 1961

hypogonadism,[1] hypospermia,[2] alopecia (certain baldness), immune disorders, skin issues, night blindness, impaired taste and wound healing.

The first signs of zinc deficiency in marginally nourished children are slow growth, anorexia, and impaired taste.[3] Pioneering medical doctors of the last century, believed that if a condition is due to malnourishment, prescription drugs cure it.

The number one source of zinc in the American diet is beef. Only three ounces provides 40% of the amount most people need daily. A deficiency occurs in vegetarians also because of their high copper diet heavy in whole grains, beans, and nuts,[4] which opposes zinc. Combined with the absence of high zinc foods of meat, eggs, liver, and poultry, it can be a problem.

A copper imbalance can lead to fatigue, and is associated with cancer of estrogen-affected organs. Estrogen dominance and high copper are associated with infertility. Zinc deficiency is also associated with compromised immunity (frequent colds and infections), depression, and poor appetite. Right ratios are the key here, as with other minerals and trace minerals.

Most whole grain breads have phytin that prevents absorption of minerals, including zinc. The phytin of sour dough bread may have been neutralized. This was the bread of Bible times except at the Feast of Unleavened Bread. Whole grain kernels should be soaked 24 hours before cooking on low temperatures. Soy products, a staple for vegans, interfere with zinc absorption more than any other mineral.[5]

Alpha-Lipoic Acid (ALA) works in the body's mitochondria "powerhouses" to assist in energy production. Its action as an antioxidant is powerful because it works on both water and fat-soluble free radicals. It protects the liver, prevents cataracts,

---

[1] Sex glands produce little or no hormones.
[2] Low semen volume does not provide medium for sperm to reach wife's cervix, common cause of infertility.
[3] http://www.merck.com/mrkshared/mmanual/section1/chapter4/4e.jsp
[4] Sesame seeds, macadamia nuts, and green pumpkin seeds, all have a good zinc:copper balance.
[5] Most zinc is lost in processing, or exists in small amounts due to depleted soils; hence many Americans may be deficient, whether vegetarians or not.

enhances immune function, and may slow Alzheimer's disease progression. Every cell in our bodies requires this critical, sulfur-containing fatty acid, chiefly to generate energy to keep us alive and functioning well.

It is also vital for bodily energy-producing reactions that convert blood sugar to energy. It is thought to prevent, and used to treat, many age-related diseases. These include diabetic neuropathy (nerve-damaged extremities) and other diabetic complications, as well as other heart disease, stroke and cataracts. Highest sources are red meat muscle, heart, and liver.

Disturbing Deficiencies Disclosure!

Low levels of quite a number of vital nutrients were discovered when adherents of a vegan diet were surveyed. To the foundation's credit, the results were posted at that website for quite sometime. Supplementation plus green barley and other powders, have been added to the diet; however, animal-based foods, chief components of God's plan for eating after Eden,[1] may have supplied all but one or two of the deficient nutrients. Here are those results as posted.

Protein: very low at 0.66g/kg of body weight. Even the FDA recommends 0.80g/kg. Since proteins catalyze all the reactions in our bodies' cells, and control virtually all cellular processes, this is a particularly troublesome matter. Participants in the study ate only 4% protein, 24% fats, and a whopping 72% of the calories as carbs. A diet with better balance of the macronutrients might be healthier and more satisfying for most. To prevent weight gain with the high carb level, breakfast consists of green powder; there is a scant lunch, and carbs are chiefly restricted to one meal.

Interestingly, approximately **60%** of those in the survey, said they ate an average of 29 grams/day of *animal-based protein* in spite of a very high 18 servings/day of fruits and vegetables - even though animal-based products are a "strictly prohibited category of foods in this diet." Actually, those who eat meat are *not* vegans. More than half those surveyed, did not "walk their talk."

---

[1] Vit. C complex is found in raw meat; however, the Bible tells us to cook our meat.

While the leaders call this "cheating," the Bible calls it hypocrisy, common among vegans as noted in 1 Timothy 4:1. I have witnessed first hand the same "cheating" in another vegetarian cult. It seems to be part of the "territory" that comes with such diets in general.

Though 29 grams/day of protein is not an adequate amount of animal-based food, it may also indicate that more than half those surveyed, were searching for satiety. On the other hand, Psalm 103:5 reminds us that the Creator's plan for eating is filling and satisfying.

A very high number of servings were consumed by survey participants, likely due to hunger. From the posted deficiencies, it is unlikely many kinds of organic fruits and vegetables were consumed. (Organic foods have been shown to contain significantly higher levels of nutrients.) A variety of foods is necessary to provide many different nutrients to nourish different tissues and organs. That does not mean a wide variety of plant foods every day so that there is no room for nutrient-dense foods, including meats, yogurt, sauerkraut, and broth.

What we want to avoid is limiting vegetable/fruit consumption to the same few daily, e.g. potatoes, carrots, lettuce, and tomatoes, with perhaps an apple thrown in for good measure. God created a host of different fruits and vegetables with varying nutrients in each, depending upon the soil and how they are handled after harvesting. We must first include the nutrient-dense, animal-based foods, and secondly, dark green, red, and yellow plant foods higher in phytonutrients.

Amazingly, the analysis published at the web site, concluded first that this dietary pattern of food choices and timing of eating, allows a low calorie diet that is adequate "in most nutrients" [!] without the need to restrict the amount of [allowed] food eaten, howbeit "...when implemented and supplemented carefully..." Even if a diet were adequate – and clearly this one is not - how many followers are capable or willing to implement or supplement it carefully, for an indefinite period of time?

Dean Esmay and his wife worked extremely hard at following a vegan diet of high carbs, low fats, and low protein in order to heal their many ailments, particularly stabilization of blood sugar. The more carefully they followed the vegan diet, the more fatigued and sicker they became, Esmay wrote. He would awaken in the middle of the night actually "aching with hunger" though they were eating huge amounts of allowed foods. The Esmay's escape from veganism bondage, with a radical, rapid turn around with animal-based foods, is exciting to read! A visit to that web site could be educational and beneficial.[1]

Vitamin B complex: B_{12}, niacin, biotin, and pantothenic acid were all reported deficient in the survey. Vitamin B is considered to be the most deficient vitamin in the US, and apparently the HD is not the solution. Water soluble and therefore not stored in the body, Vitamin B is involved with heart nourishment, neurological disorders, metabolism of macronutrients, endurance, energy, handling of stress, bodily production of steroids, adrenal support, fighting allergies, mental health, anxiety, and depression; water retention, weight gain and loss, and much other. This complex of eight catalysts, mostly works in synergism.

A diet void of animal-based foods would contain no vitamin B_{12} since plant foods have none bioavailable to humans. Because this vital nutrient is required for DNA, protecting the nervous system, and producing blood cells, mankind would not have long lived after the fall without animal-based foods as we have shown.

There is absolutely no evidence, either scriptural or scientific, that "...in Biblical times, plants contained B_{12} absorbed from the soil." It is very likely that before the Fall, man's body produced adequate B_{12}.

Vitamin D: deficiency of this critical nutrient among survey participants, reflected the typical vegan population.

Calcium: Even if the vegan diet could provide adequate calcium, it does not provide required nutrients for calcium absorption. A former vegan testified that while his family was eating this way, his baby cut his first tooth - with most of the enamel missing. The other teeth came in completely normal after raw goat milk was added to the baby's diet.[2]

---

[1] beyondveg.com/cat/frank-talk/index.shtml
[2] Foote, A., *Vegan Diet Deficiencies Injure Baby: Our Experience with Deficiencies of the **HD***

Only two of the survey participants were not seriously deficient in their calcium intake. The present RDI is more than double the intake. Even if calcium intake had been adequate, protein, and many other nutrients are required for the absorption of this mineral, as explained.

Though B_{12} was added to this diet a few years before; B_{12}, plus calcium and vitamin D, were low for almost everyone in the 2001 survey. Adequate cholesterol is important for the skin's ability to absorb sunlight for the latter nutrient. Only animal-based foods supply dietary cholesterol.

Vitamin C: The mean daily intake was estimated to be 329 mg. since an ascorbic acid supplement was taken which skewed results of the actual amount. Ascorbic acid is only the "outer shell" of the vitamin C complex. Vitamin C is important for iron absorption. Interestingly, this nutrient is found in meat that is not overly cooked, as proven by Dr. V. Stefansson's all meat diet. We obtain vitamin C complex from whole foods and whole-foods concentrates.

Selenium works in tandem with vitamin E. This trace mineral is needed in very small amounts for antioxidants, thyroid function, and immune system. It's deficiency has been identified in asthma patients.

Iron from animal products (heme), especially liver, red meat, and dark meat of poultry, is easily absorbed, whereas iron from fruits, vegetables, grains, and supplements (non-heme), is difficult to absorb. A high fiber diet may also inhibit iron absorption. Anemia is a common risk for vegans. More about fiber later.

Zinc was also low in the participants. Its importance cannot be overestimated. Found everywhere in the body, it functions in a broad range, is critical for many of our bodily systems, including the immune system for infection resistance. It is involved in wound healing, and in cell growth and division where it is important for protein and DNA synthesis, obviously no small matter. The liver needs it to function, and it is important for insulin activity.

Our muscles use 60% of the body's supply, the bones 30%, and skin 5%. This trace mineral is very important for reproductive organs, female ovaries and male prostate (the more sexually active the man is, the more zinc he will require; semen contains 100 times more zinc than the blood). Zinc is not stored in the body. An adequate daily intake is vital. A vital component of myriad enzymes, it is also required for dietary protein, carb and fat processing by the body.

High dietary fiber and phytic acid inhibit zinc absorption. They are found in whole-grain cereals, nuts, beans and peas. Their adverse effects on zinc absorption can be diminished by pre-soaking these foods for 24 hours. However, whole grains and legumes, often high in vegan diets, were surprisingly low in this group's dietary intake. Hence we might assume that the zinc deficiency is due to inhibiting phytates in soy products, though protein was low also. This is one serious consequence of bypassing God's plan for eating after the Fall.

Vitamin A: Remember, real vitamin A comes from animal-based foods. The provitamin, beta carotene, which vegans take for this, cannot be converted to vitamin A by some people. Vitamins A, D, E, and K require fat for absorption.

God's nutrients work best synergistically, in the food, rather than as fractionated isolates in pill form.[1] Besides quality protein, vitamins and minerals, animal-based foods provide fatty acids and other very important properties, e.g. the X-Factor[2] and CLA. We do not know how many more nutrients and phytochemicals have yet to be discovered.

Digestive Weakness

Fifty percent of our population has digestive issues, medical literature declares. Worse than Adam's after the Fall, today's digestive problems are pandemic – from our infants to the aging. This is said to be the #1 problem for which Americans seek medical attention in the new millenium.

---

[1] The next best form is whole foods concentrates. See Resources.
[2] We will discuss this recently identified nutrient in Chapter 9.

Not only does the post-Eden life require more nourishment due to inferior digestion, the Sad American Diet (SAD) itself does not support but opposes a healthy digestive system necessary for vitamin B_{12} absorption. Often when patients eat only God's nutritious foods, beginning with small amounts of quality meat and other flesh foods, digestion normalizes. The principle here is that when we stop doing that which causes the problem and begin providing the body what it needs (increased quality and variety of nutrients), it heals itself.

Rejuvenation!

A favorite client and registered nurse, was a sarcoma victim who had been unable to eat animal-source foods for three and one-half years subsequent to extended chemotherapy. She suffered chronic stomach pain, indigestion, and lactose intolerance. Her inability to sleep more than three or so hours each night was most stressful. Most of one thigh had been surgically removed after incredible radiation treatments requiring hospitalization after each. A year later the femur bone snapped and a rod was inserted. After a second break a longer rod replaced the first.

Confined to a wheelchair, she attended a large conference where I spoke about osteoporosis. I didn't see her at that time; was unaware that she was unable to get up to the podium before I had to leave.

I was to begin work on these books before that city-sponsored conference, and had asked the Lord not to allow anyone to call afterward except whom He wanted me to work with as I was not taking new patients. The next week this petite shell of a woman called me requesting help with her chiefly carbohydrate vegan diet. I agreed to do what I could by way of telephone consults.

First I had her discontinue her multiple mineral supplement with a very long list of inorganic ingredients. I then had her change her diet to fresh, whole foods the Creator designed for her body. Right away the stomach pain ceased. She was very pleased.

She called every few days, very excited to report how increasingly good she already felt. Soon she was sleeping all night again. However, she remained very fearful of animal protein. It was very difficult for this vegan to gradually add meat, fish, poultry, and eggs to her diet. Yet she was highly motivated and compliant.

We began with an ounce of lightly cooked organic beef liver with breakfast, and an ounce or two of fresh salmon for lunch along with fresh, lightly steamed vegetables. I also had her properly balance the protein, carbs, and right fats for her needs. Then we added raw goat cheese, raw milk and butter, teaching her to make her own raw yogurt. Her husband was ecstatic! He had been very concerned about her lack of animal protein, and failing health.

Medical monitoring continued as we gradually introduced a protocol of whole-foods concentrates and a couple of herbs; all nutritionally supporting appetite, digestion, bone building, immune system, liver, and enhancing wellness overall. Within a few weeks after she first called she was out of the wheelchair and walking with a cane. Then she added resistance exercise.

Three months after I began working with this patient, she attended a lecture and introduced herself. What vim and vigor! She was absolutely radiant!

Having returned to the work she loves, today this fifty-five year old is a powerful testimony of the amazing restoration our magnificent "healing machines" were designed to achieve. After removal of one of the deadliest cancers, years of radical treatments of toxic drugs, intensive chemo and irradiation, as well as the deficient vegan diet, when she provided her body quality, animal-based foods required for healing, it did just that within a remarkably short time.

And What Of Lacto-Ovo Vegetarians?

Lacto-ovo vegetarians do not eat meat, fish or poultry, usually because death to animals is required. However, they include eggs and dairy products in their diets. If whole, organic foods are consumed, this can be fairly healthy, especially if eggs are eaten in adequate amounts from pastured hens, and dairy products are from grass-fed cows. Rarely is this the case. Most often, ultrapasteurized skim milk, low-fat, artificial cheese, soy-fed hens' eggs, and high carbs are the food sources for this group.

Our bodies can metabolize only so much protein daily, thus we must get other calories from fat and carbs. Therefore, if we consume a low fat diet, we must depend heavily upon carbs as vegans do. Studies show a high carb diet is involved with atherosclerosis, diabetes, and other serious conditions.[1] Right fats are important as blood sugar stabilizers for high carbs, especially refined foods with simple carbs. High consumption of Omega 6 vegetable oils has been associated with cancer, and blood clots leading to MI. Eggs and whole milk provide healthy fats that are not rancid or nutrient deficient, and do not require antioxidants.

Ovo-vegetarians (eggs only) who eat thus for ethical reasons, try to avoid fertilized eggs and caviar (made from fish eggs), because they involve deaths of the chick embryo and pregnant fish. Never mind that in order to provide eggs, the commercial farmers kill half the chicks hatched for layers, i.e., the males. Some say that is ovo-vegetarian hypocrisy, and inconsistent at the least.

And where is the vegetarian conviction in eating cheese, sour cream, drinking milk, and eating yogurt, when cows must produce calves every year in order stay "fresh" (produce milk) and be profitable? Like the chicks, approximately half the calves are males, few of which are kept for breeding, the rest are killed. Yet most people who eat "lacto-vegetarian," don't eat meat because it involves killing. Again, is that not hypocrisy, and inconsistent at the least?

Like other wellness practitioners, I find that most vegetarians are self-deceived, including lacto-ovo advocates; believing they are actually well nourished even when their blood work may show something different. As my colleagues also observe, some vegetarians don't believe test results, and attempt to convince me vegetarianism is best for the human race.

Dr. Airola's Death-Dealing Diet

In his book, *Worldwide Secrets for Staying Young* (1982), Paavo Airola, ND, PhD, claimed to offer "proven and effective ways to halt and reverse the aging processes, and live a long and healthy life." A massive stroke killed him one year later at age 64.

---

[1] Allan B, Lutz W, *Life Without Bread,* Keats, 2000

Everyone of the first 13 chapters of that book, provides "health and longevity secrets" from far and wide. (Dr. Airola directed biological medical clinics in Mexico and Europe.) In this volume, the misguided doctor expressed his conviction that humans should live to be 120 years old, barring killing themselves prematurely "by violating the basic laws of health and life." Ironically, he did broke one of the chief "laws of health and life."

The 120 years seems to be the life span vegetarians, and especially vegans aspire to, whether Christian or non-Christian. That "magic number" has been bandied around among the Hallelujah Diet movement as well. It is claimed that vegetarian Norman Walker, DSc., lived almost 120 years, though official records show 99 years, no small fete in itself, certainly not nearly 120.

With Christians, some believe "…My Spirit shall not always strive with man…yet his days shall be a hundred and twenty years," refers to man's new life span, beginning before the flood in Genesis 6:3. The 120 figure may arise from that misinterpretation where God gave the wicked people 120 years to repent while Noah preached to them and built the ark.

Dr. Airola was an internationally known vegetarian following more closely veganism. He was a physician, author, and renowned lecturer. He occasionally drank raw goat milk. Dr. Airola taught that

> …our actual daily need of protein is 30-40 grams…**even less if raw protein from milk and vegetable sources are used**…Almonds, sesame seeds, soybeans, buckwheat, peanuts, sunflower seeds, pumpkin seeds, potatoes, and all leafy green vegetables contain **complete proteins,** which are comparable in quality to animal proteins…[emphases in the original].

Of this list, only soy and buckwheat contain complete protein, yet they are not of the quality of clean animal protein, and do not offer those important fats.

There was kindness and good character manifested in Dr. Airola's writings. And there were some good things about the Airola philosophy and teaching – as far as it went. However, he believed meat caused cancer. Unfortunately, in demeaning most of the Creator's animal-based, nutrient-dense foods, he deprived himself of that which his body urgently required in order to fulfill even his allotted 70 years.

With Japan's lean diet and low cholesterol, more people die from cerebral hemorrhage (stroke). Solid science supports the principle of the necessity for animal-based foods for human dietary intake, for a number of reasons. Unfortunately, in refusing all these but eggs and sometimes milk, Dr. Airola also rejected one of the most important of God's dietary health laws. The doctor lived only half the time he was sure he would.

Nutritional deficiencies and imbalances may go on for years before the evidence begins to manifest in symptoms of nutritional-related disease. In the US, the risk of cerebral hemorrhage is high for those with low cholesterol combined with elevated blood pressure.[1] We have personal knowledge of another vegan leader rushed to the hospital for emergency care. He too suffered a hemorrhagic stroke, and high blood pressure. Are the "emperor's news clothes" wearing thin?

MULTIPLE MYTHS OF VEGETARIANSIM

1. Carnivores, Herbivores & Omnivores – Which Are You?

In order to know which is the proper diet, we must settle an important question: to which of these three groups does man belong? With respect to the anatomy of humans, understanding is usually flawed. We are told repeatedly and often that man's digestive system was not created for meat eating, only vegetarianism, specifically veganism.[2]

As an anatomist and a primatologist, John McArdle, PhD, is a former scientific advisor to The American Anti-Vivisection Society. Dr. McArdle speaks with authority with respect to the misinformation regarding man's supposedly naturally being a vegetarian:

---

[1] Ravnskov U, *The Cholesterol Myths, Exposing the Falacy That Sat. Fat & Chol. Cause Heart Disease,* p.240

[2] Medical schools now include anatomy only in specialists courses, rather than for all medical doctors.

There are a number of popular myths about vegetarianism that have no scientific basis in fact. One of these myths is that man is naturally a vegetarian because our bodies resemble plant eaters, not carnivores. In fact we are omnivores, capable of either eating meat or plant foods. The following addresses the unscientific theory of man being only a plant eater.

> Much of the misinformation on the issue of man's being a natural vegetarian arises from confusion between taxonomic (in biology, the procedure of classifying organisms in established categories) and dietary characteristics...
>
> The key category in the discussion of human diet is omnivores, which are defined as generalized feeders, with neither carnivore nor herbivore specializations for acquiring or processing food, and who are capable of consuming and do consume both animal protein and vegetation...
>
> As far back as it can be traced, clearly the archeological record indicates an omnivorous diet for humans that included meat...Once domestication of food sources began, it included both animals and plants."[1]

That is my own view as well; i.e., once outside Eden when man began producing his own food, his diet became omnivorous, as mentioned.

As an expert in the study of primates, Dr. McArdle further explains that the smallest primates eat insects exclusively. The largest are vegetarians. Only the latter eat a pure vegetarian diet, the remaining primates in between have

---

[1] As published by the Vegetarian Resource Group, Baltimore, MD. http://www.vrg.org/nutshell/omni.htm

> "...dietary preferences that reflect the daily food intake needs of each body size and the relative availability of food resources in a tropical forest...[Chimps]...frequently kill and eat other mammals (including other primates)...Nearly all plant eaters have fermenting vats (enlarged chambers [in the body] where food sits and microbes attack it)...Humans have no such specializations.

Another critical point which denies man is intended to eat vegan, is that he normally produces large amounts of hydrochloric acid in his stomach, undesirable for digesting plant foods only, which are chiefly alkaline.

2. The Myth Of The Digestive Track Length: Where Does It End?

Vegetarians often refer to the length of the human GI tract in an attempt to prove man should not eat meat. However, explains Dr. McArdle,

> Relative number and distribution of cell types, as well as structural specializations, are more important than overall length of the intestine in determining a typical diet.

With the carnivore's high level of stomach acid, raw meat is easy for them to digest; thus they have short intestines.[1] In contrast, plant material is more difficult to digest and therefore herbivores tend to have long intestines (or multiple stomachs), which prolong the digestive process. Omnivores, such as humans, have intestines of moderate length to digest both plants and flesh foods. If our Creator intended us to consume a pure vegan diet, why then did He design human anatomy to digest both plants and meats?

---

[1] These animals swallow their raw food without chewing, and have high levels of stomach acid to digest meat. Many Americans may have inadequate levels of stomach acid today, and meat is prepared so as to denature it, making the digestion of protein difficult. A qualified natural physician can assist with appropriate digestive modalities.

Another speculation is that God commanded Noah to eat meat when he came off the ark because all vegetation had been destroyed by the flood. Yet the dove found green growth (*before* Noah left the ark) necessary for the animals who didn't eat meat, and for man.

In fact, God specifically commanded Noah to eat meat together with green plants, when he disembarked from the ark.[1] We see God's *meat and greens mentioned together* again in Psalm 104:14, repeating the fact of the omnivorous anatomy of man.

> He causes the grass to grow for the cattle, and herbs[2] for the service of man; that he may bring forth food out of the earth.

Grass and then cattle predigest earth's minerals and trace minerals for us. As this text states, through these (and other plants and clean animals) we receive sustenance directly and indirectly from the earth from which man came.

A number of Christian vegans are taking their faulty understanding of the human anatomy to perilous conclusions. If we reject truth, we may ultimately embrace a lie.[3] This particular deception has become a five-part delusion as follows:

1. God designed humans as vegetarians to digest only plants.
2. He then "permitted" humans to eat meat.
3. Because meat has no fiber, it sits in the bowel and putrefies.
4. The meat rotting in the bowel causes terrible diseases.
5. These diseases drastically reduce man's life span, *God's intention.*

---

[1] Eating meat was not a temporary provision for Noah since 1 Timothy 4 speaks of eating meat in latter times.

[2] Heb. *eh-seb*, tender green shoots, the same Heb. word in both Gen. 1:29, 30, and 9:3.

[3] 2 Thes. 2:11

Based upon fundamental errors in reasoning, these fallacious five points are filled with the wisdom of man, and disbelief of the clear Word of God. They favor bad science and demonstrate a lack of knowledge.

Error is truth taken to the extreme, e.g., these vegans teach that since meat has no fiber, you should not eat meat at all, only fibrous foods.[1] When God told us to eat meat, He well knew it contains no fiber; *at the same* time, He told us to eat plants along with it. Yet fiber is not the whole story, as we'll see.

The present diseases of the GI track did not exist before America's highly processed foods were stripped of nutrients. White flour, white sugar, white shortening, white rice, and white French fries are most favored ingredients, with the latter being the only vegetable many Americans consume. All these are constipating, preventing the movement of whatever is in the bowel, including meat. Fiber lack is only part of it.

For both alike - those who go to the extreme of eating no meat - and those who eat meat but nothing of God's fresh, whole fruits and vegetables, it is dangerous, spiritually and physiologically. "This you ought to have done, and not left the other undone," Paul would say to both. Yet green foods include more than fiber.

3. A Tooth Is A Tooth Is A Tooth? *The* Big Difference

The best evidence as to whether animals or humans are omnivorous comes not from the gut, but from dentition (teeth). There are distinct differences in the teeth of carnivores (meat eaters), herbivores (plant eaters), and omnivores (eaters of both meat and plants). We learn in college biology that

> Mammalian tooth patterns are interesting because <u>no other vertebrate has different kinds of teeth within one individual</u>. In the front of the mouth are incisors, teeth that function in ripping or chiseling. On each side of the incisors may be found the canines, useful in biting and piercing prey. Behind the canines are the cheek teeth: the

---

[1] Too much fiber is not healthy.

premolars, that do some grinding, and the molars, that do most of the grinding and chewing...[1]

Hence humans are biologically suited for an omnivorous diet including flesh and plant foods, unlike herbivores and carnivores. The former have flat teeth (cattle, sheep, goats), and the latter pointed teeth (lions, tigers, wolves).

As with the digestive track, again we must ask ourselves, if the Creator intended humans to eat only plant foods, why did He give man teeth to chew both plant and flesh foods?

4. Man's Gallbladder: Cut It Out & Ignore It?

Another anatomical feature of carnivores (meat eaters) and omnivores is the gallbladder, which distinguishes between these and herbivores. Man's gallbladder stores large amounts of detergent bile for enhancing digestion and breaking down fats into fatty acids so they can be absorbed. Animals which do not eat meat, have no gallbladders, as the liver alone quickly supplies adequate bile.[2]

Other Mundane Myths

There are countless other myths associated with vegetarianism. They range from "Eating meat is inhumane, causes osteoporosis, cancer" and you name it, to "Meat consumption contributes to famine and depletes the earth's natural resources." Some of those myths are debunked in this book in-depth, however, it would require another book to deal with them all.

Not to worry, there is a splendid website called *Nexus, The Myths of Vegetarianism,* that addresses at least fifteen issues of this misinformation at its website.[3] The documentation is scientific and sound. Be sure and visit *Nexus.*

---

[1] Biology 105-106, Cornell Univ.
[2] Fats stimulate the gallbladder to empty itself. Low fat diets allow the bile to stagnate in the gallbladder.
[3] nexusmagazine.com/articles/vegemyths1.html#34

Millions of Americans are avoiding fats for fear of CVD. While it is true high blood triglycerides are associated with these diseases, these fats do not come from dietary saturated fats. We have been taught for half a century to eat high carbs. High carbs, especially processed, simple ones, e.g., white flour and refined sugar - are handled by the liver as excess, unused glucose; and converted to triglycerides. Ironically, it is this fat that is then deposited on bellies and thighs as *saturated* fat!

Human Anatomy Does Not Support A Vegetarian Diet

Plainly and precisely, Dr. McArdle determines that

> Humans are classic examples of omnivores in all relevant anatomical traits. There is no basis in anatomy or physiology for the assumption that humans are pre-adapted to the vegetarian diet.[1]

In Conclusion

Vegetarianism is neither scientifically nor scripturally sound. It is a deviation from God's whole menu, His nutritional best for man since the Fall. In the next chapter we will take a close look at some amazing vegan examples history has provided for our further learning.

---

[1] vrg.org/nutshell/omni.htm, *Vegetarianism In A Nutshell,* a vegan website

9

Veganism – Many "Spins" Same Sin

Mahatma Gandhi's Fraud & Failure

Father of the Nation, India's Gandhi, was adamantly opposed to animal-based foods. However, after a lifetime of attempting to successfully eat a vegan diet, the Hindu leader confessed it was not possible to do so and be healthy; and that vegan claims to the contrary were fraudulent. Arnold DeVries, an anthropologist, wrote at length concerning Gandhi's dietary struggle. DeVries' most revealing commentary included the following:

> The late Mahatma Gandhi devoted much of his life to the advocacy of a strict vegetarian diet, and for years he experimented on his own body to find a suitable selection of plant foods on which to sustain health. But all attempts were failures. In 1929, Gandhi and 22 companions went on a diet consisting of a limited selection of uncooked plant foods. Whereas the diet worked out well **for a time** and led to marked improvement in consumptive [TB] cases, it failed to prove adequate on a **long-range** sustenance basis. One by one Gandhi's companions were forced to depart from the diet, and Gandhi himself had to add goat milk to his fare in order to regain [his strength].
>
> "For my companions I have been a *blind guide leading the blind*," declared Gandhi after the experiment was over. Gandhi still felt, however, that "...the hidden

possibilities of the innumerable seeds, leaves and fruits..." of the earth could be explored and found to provide mankind with adequate nourishment. He never stopped trying to experiment along these lines, but he always had to turn back to goat milk to regain his strength. In the end he had to acknowledge the necessity for animal[-based] food. In 1946 he declared:

> The scores of India today get neither milk nor ghee nor butter, nor even buttermilk. No wonder that mortality figures are on the increase and there is a **lack of energy** in the people. It would appear as if man is really unable to sustain life without either meat or milk, and milk products. Anyone who deceives people in this regard or countenances the fraud,[1] is an enemy of India.[2]

Further wrote DeVries:

> These are strong words from a man who devoted most of his life to the search for a satisfactory vegetarian diet. But Gandhi's experience is not unique in the field of nutrition. Many others have also gone through the experience of believing that man could thrive exclusively upon a limited selection of uncooked plant foods, only to find in the end that animal products were necessary for sustenance...

As you review further profiles of some of veganism's leaders, see if you can identify some common traits found among them all, be they Christian or no.

Vegan/Prophetess Ellen G. White

Founder of the Seventh Day Adventist Church, vegan Ellen G. White, had a difficult time not eating animal-based foods she publicly denounced and demanded members of her church avoid.

---

[1] "Speaking lies in hypocrisy..." 1 Tim. 4:2 has it.
[2] DeVries, A, *The Elixir of Life,* 1952. Milk alone is not adequate for optimum health long-term.

Here are some statements evidencing that long period of inconsistency.[1]

1869:

I have not changed my course a particle since I adopted the health reform. I have not taken one step back since the light from heaven upon this subject first shone upon my pathway. I broke away from everything at once, from meat and butter, and from three meals. I left off those things from principle. I took my stand on health reform from principle.[2]

No butter or flesh-meats of any kind come on my table.[3]

Eggs should not be placed upon your table. They are an injury to your children.[4]

1873:

A young man from Nova Scotia had come in from hunting. He had a quarter of deer...He gave us a small piece of the meat, which we made into broth. Willie shot a duck which came in a time of need, for our supplies were rapidly diminishing.[5]

1882:

Mary, if you can get me a good box of herrings, fresh ones, please do so. These last ones that Willie got are bitter and old...if you can get a few cans of good oysters, get them.[6]

1890s:

Prominent surgeon John Kellogg, of Battle Creek, Michigan, a Seventh-Day Adventist member, and founder of the

---

[1] We are indebted to Dr. Michel E. Todd for his comprehensive, orderly compilation of these facts as provided at biblebelievers.com/sda/sda3./html#3-
[2] Testimonies to the church, Vol. 2, pp. 371-372
[3] Testimonies, Vol. 2, p. 487
[4] Testimonies, Volume 2, p. 400
[5] Ms. 11, 1873. Released by the Ellen G. White Estate, Wash, D.C., April 11, 1985; MR 14, p.353
[6] Ltr. to daughter-in-law, Mary White, May 31, 1882, from Healdsburg, CA

luxurious Battle Creek Sanitarium and health club,[1] declared that when Mrs. White visited the sanitarium in the 1890s, she "always called for meat and usually fried chicken," which bothered Dr. Kellogg no little bit since he was a vegetarian.

Dr. Kellogg also recalled hearing the Whites' young son, Edson (J.E.), calling out to the meat wagon while standing in front of the family tent at a church camp meeting, "'Say, hello there! Have you any fresh fish?" 'No,' was his reply. "Have you got any fresh chicken?' Again the answer was 'No,' and J.E. bawled out in a very loud voice, 'Mother wants some chicken. You had better get some quick!'"[2]

Seventh-Day Adventist president A.G. Daniels, and his wife Mary, lived with the Whites for sometime. In 1919, four years after Mrs. White's death, speaking at a conference, Mr. Daniels said, "I have eaten pounds of butter at her table myself, and dozens of eggs."

Also, some years after Mrs. White's death, another son, Willie, told of his mother's great difficulty in giving up her meat. He recalled "lunch baskets filled with turkey, chicken, and tinned tongue."[3]

It is said that Mrs. White finally did quit eating meat in January 1894. Strangely, it was not for spiritual reasons or because of the "angels who spoke" to her, but for animal rights. She explained:

> ...But when the selfishness of taking the lives of animals to gratify a perverted taste was presented to me by a Catholic woman, kneeling at my feet, I felt ashamed and distressed. I saw it in a new light, and I said, "I will no longer patronize the butchers. I will not have the flesh of corpses on my table."[4]

The eating of not only meat but unclean meat and seafood, e.g., pork and oysters, was likewise confusing to H. E. Carver, an

---

[1] geocities.com/Athens/oracle/9840/kellogg.html as viewed Feb. 19, 2007 (excellent article)
[2] Kellogg ltr to Ballenger, Jan 9, 1936
[3] Prophetess of Health, pp. 171-171
[4] Spalding & Magan, p.38

early Adventists, who witnessed contradicting responses from Mr. and Mrs. White, and Mrs. White herself.[1] Finally, there is this disturbing message to the church from her:

> Let not any of our ministers set an **evil example** in the eating of flesh-meat. Let them and their families live up to the light of health reform. Let not our ministers **animalize their own nature and the nature of their children.**"[2]

Dear reader, not only was the "water muddied" by the conflicting responses from Mrs. White, but ostensibly, she previously had written a letter rebuking a church member who felt eating pork was wrong.[3]

It would seem the last of Mrs. White's response above, hinges on serious sacrilege. Did God set an "evil example" in eating meat before Abraham and Sarah?

And what of Jesus' example in preparing fish and eating this, lamb, and doubtless other meat He created for this and listed in His Word?[4] Worst of all, what of the "animalizing" of His "...own nature and the nature of [His] children,"[5] to say nothing of God's commandments to His children to eat meat, blessed by Him. Did such admonition come from the God of the Bible?

New Age Aim: Return To Genesis 1:29

Just as some Christian vegans seek to return to the Genesis 1:29 diet, so too do some New Age churches. In the forthright account that follows, we have a compelling example of another former vegan national leader who, like Gandhi and many others, desperately wanted the vegan diet to work.

---

[1] See biblebelievers.com/SDA/SDA3.html#3-d for details
[2] Spalding & Magan, p.211
[3] See biblebelievers.com/SDA/SDA3.html#3-d for details.
[4] Lev. 11, 14; 1 Tim. 4:3
[5] Some Christian vegans claim that Jesus did not eat meat before He received His glorified body. We find no reason or Scripture for that position.

The website doctrinal statement of the New Age Essene Church of Christ (NAECC), declares that we are entering "a new age of relatively advanced spirituality," in which "the **group consciousness** takes a quantum leap forward."[1] According to this religion, Isaiah prophesied a non-violent, vegetarian civilization, "returning to the original non-flesh diet given by God in Genesis." (The Genesis 1:29 diet of the authorized Bible was not only vegetarian, but vegan. It included no animal-source foods whatever.)

The NAECC includes vegetarianism as "an absolute requirement of discipleship" and "the only proof" that it is "the restored church of the Essene Master Jesus" and "his lost teachings, including his doctrine on vegetarianism." Based upon "another gospel"[2] and "another Jesus," the NAECC teaches that "Vegetarianism was **REQUIRED** by Jesus of any person who wanted to become his disciple." (Emphasis in the original.)

Lying Hypocrites, Seared Consciences

In Canadian vegan F. Patenaude's interview with Nazariah, national leader and pastor of the above mentioned New Age church, Nazariah frankly tells of his five years on a raw vegan diet, at which time he completely "…lost the ability to walk" and was literally paralyzed with pain in all his extremeties. His hands, fingers, and feet were in such pain he could not move, he says.

Further, Nazariah states he experienced central nervous system problems, and severe catabolism (in which the body consume its muscles for complete protein). "Five years on the vegan diet resulted in my body falling apart," he informed the vegan culture. He says he healed himself with the addition of cultured raw dairy products and eggs to supply vitamin B_{12} and complete protein. As did Gandhi, he now preaches, "In the short term, you don't have those sorts of problems. They're nutritional deficiencies that take several years to manifest themselves."

As you read on, you will understand why many vegan leaders struggle with deception and hypocrisy. Nazariah is to be highly

---

[1] As viewed Oct. 7, 2006 at essene.org/Essene_Doctrine.htm#Doctrine_five.
[2] Gal. 1:6-9

commended for his courageous candor and service to mankind in the very revealing 2004 interview published on the Internet at a number of web sites after his very serious health issues. Having openly confessed his mistake, and added cultured yogurt and eggs to his diet, Nazariah's forthright report exposes veganism's inherent "speaking lies in hypocrisy..." with seared conscience, as Scripture describes it.[1]

Nazariah told of his previous great zeal for veganism, and whenever he heard other vegans describe health issues attributed to the diet, he was certain they were either detoxifying or were not following the diet correctly.[2] Then his own serious health problems led to a more enlightened perspective.

As a regular speaker at raw-food events, this pastor "hung out" with other such notable leaders, was often at their homes, got to know them well. Soon he discovered that the conditions he had suffered, "...were **rampant** in the raw-vegan movement, but don't get talked about." (The same is sometimes true in the Christian vegan community.) Leaders of that movement are experiencing anxiety attacks, panic attacks, clinical depression, joint pain, muscle loss, tooth loss, and other problems, reported this pastor. However, what was most troubling was that *they didn't want their admiring public to know.*

Time after time, an ailing deceiver called Nazariah for "...advice for dealing with these ailments," he disclosed. But "at the very next big, raw food conference, there that person would be, preaching the amazing benefits of the 100% raw vegan diet, signing copies of their books, and speaking negatively about cooked food eaters, and those who eat only partially raw, or are not vegan." The awareness of the many leaders' deceiving their devoted, trusting followers, "stung" the pastor like a scorpion.

---

[1] The entire interview was viewed at fredericpatenaude.com/articles/interview-nazariah.html. Nazariah graciously offered us a hard copy.

[2] "When doctors don't know what's wrong, they blame the patient," a nationally known medical school dept. head once told us. And so too, this is the most common response when veganism doesn't work.

Not Just A Religion, But A Living

This rare, courageous leader revealed to the world that when the lecturers and authors of books about the "perfect diets" of veganism " begin experiencing health issues associated with the diet, they "...hide the fact, because they are earning their livings being raw-food lecturers/authors..."

He's encountered again and again, Nazariah declares, that when well known vegan leaders that he knows personally, are experiencing the conditions noted above; and he sees them speaking at raw-food conventions, "...[T]hey never mention any of the problems they're actually experiencing. They just praise how perfect the raw food vegan diet is...anytime people are having problems on the raw vegan diet," they are told they're just experiencing detox and cleansing.[1] This is nothing less than "...speaking lies with hypocrisy, having their own conscience seared with a hot iron," "...teaching things they ought not, for filthy lucre's sake." We find it often with the movement universally, Christian and non-Christian alike.

This honest discerner and pastor found that once one begins to derive their livelihood from such speaking engagements, and enjoys the "positive strokes" as an author and expert on that diet, it is "...**very hard for them to admit that the diet is not working in their own life.** It would mean that their...books were no longer valid;" they would be forced to find an honest way to make a living, he believes.

Another reason these leaders do not publicly admit their health issues with the diet is that they have been shamed into *not* admitting them. Hence each believes he is the only one suffering related health problems; it's his fault.

This former vegan says he has been in a room "...with seven raw food experts and had personal knowledge that five of them had been struggling with those problems, and yet each of them thought they were the only one." Because he was a minister, many such other leaders were comfortable seeking his counseling and confiding in him; whereas they would not mention their problems to others. (pride may enter in here as well).

---

[1] thegardendiet.com/naz.html as viewed Nov. 6, 2006.

However, it is the leaders themselves that perpetuate this shaming so that others too, believe they are the only ones experiencing failure with the seriously deficient diet. (All vegetarian/vegan diets are deficient, whether raw or partly raw.) Nazariah told of once living with several other raw food vegans. Each and every one ultimately suffered nervous disorders, and each thought he was the only one experiencing them.

One of them went on an Internet raw food message board and asked if the condition might be due to that diet; and if he should take vitamin B_{12}. In true fashion, says Nazariah, the moderator responded that "the diet is perfectly fine," that the inquirer was simply experiencing detoxification. (It is interesting that they would believe each other!)

The New Age pastor was a personal friend of the moderator and knew that the moderator himself was "...suffering from terrible panic attacks and was even considering suicide," as he had confided, "...but on the message board he moderated, he still preached the party line: all problems are just detox."

This was another clear example of 1 Timothy 4:2: "speaking lies in hypocrisy, having their own consciences seared [as with] a hot iron," caring nothing that others suffer, profiting at the expense of others' bodily decline.

Fraudulent Fry

After Nazariah's painful awakening, he read a health newsletter's detailed report of the death of the famous raw vegan, T. C. Fry.[1] I urge you, the reader, to take the time to review this absolutely incredible story as told by many contributors who had experience with this fraud. A charmer, Fry was married many times, sexually addicted, and bilked many of their money, according to reports included in the story. Claiming to eat only fruit, vegetables, nuts and seeds, some of those close to him reported seeing him eat chocolate bars and macaroni and cheese. He was "...unable to consistently follow his path that he was so successful in persuading others to follow," was Ben Russell's nice

---

[1] Day C, *Health & Beyond,* Vol. 4 Nr. 7, Nov. 1996, as viewed at http://www.chetday.com/v4n7.pdf Dec. 2006

way of saying he was a hypocrite. While we all may fall into that sin without thinking, it was a way of life for this deceiving vegan.

Fry wrote often about his "perfect health," that he had not been ill at all for decades, even when his health was failing. More than a year before this "health expert's" death, he had to have known something was seriously wrong. He actually was starving to death. Losing weight fast (about 40 pounds that year), and ematiated, he was living almost entirely on carbohydrates with few minerals. He ate no meaningful amount of protein, almost no fats.

"Colorless and ashen gray," he appeared to be about 90 years old before he was 70, wore many layers of clothing, trying to stay warm. Both feet were badly swollen with five pounds of fluids in each ankle, and he had not strength even to crawl upstairs to his bed. The primary cause of death was a coronary embolism, with multiple atherosclerotic thrombi in his lower legs, as well as a lesion in his upper left lung. Of course, the weakening fraud had difficulty breathing. He was anemic; and suffered acidosis and osteoporosis as well.

Yet while in this horrendous condition, Fry pressed on diligently to write more books on veganism, buy more ads to hawk his materials extolling his diet, going forward with plans to build a health clinic. Claiming a strong love for truth at all costs, he was actually living a large lie, never hinting at his horrid condition to any but his doctor and a few close friends.

What irony that this proud and probable contributor to the destruction of the health of many, had no tolerance for "anecdotal assertions" and "puny intellects," as he referred to reporting of diet failure from his ailing students.

A Leader Listens, Learns, & Alerts

In the same periodical in which Nazariah learned about Fry's disaster, was an article by a natural hygienist doctor who advised that these vegan diets "invariably" result in health problems. The shocking truth about Fry was followed with more disturbing deaths, one of which was closer to home.

In a nearby town, a founding member of the local vegan group dropped dead from coronary problems at a young age. The attending physician reportedly told the widow that the deceased was in an advanced stage of catabolism due to severe malnutrition that "destroyed his heart." When the widow reported back to the vegan group her husband had organized and led, she was rebuked for speaking negatively about the diet; and was told, "The doctor is wrong." They extended "the left foot of fellowship" to this new widow in deep emotional pain.

Shortly thereafter, Nazariah shared this information with a raw food vegan group leader in another state, who replied, "Oh, we just had a guy die from the very same thing. The doctors said his body had begun to eat itself due to malnutrition." I recently saw another such death report at Amazon.com book reviews, written by a grieving son whose father would not give up a popular Christian vegan diet, even though his medical doctor told him he was dying of starvation.

Nazariah stated in the interview with vegan Patenaude, that he could "go on and on reporting similar things." In other words, vegan health issues and related deaths are not uncommon known to him.

Also not surprising, this well-known former vegan (now lacto-ovo vegetarian), has found that in sharing the truth about the perils of the diet he previously zealously taught, he is getting the "brush off" with responses of disbelief. Yet he listened, and applied what he learned to save his own life, and then acted unselfishly to save the lives of many others. May his testimony here achieve more of the same.

The "Blind Leading The Blind"

Gandhi confessed and lamented this about himself and other vegan leaders. 1 Timothy 4:1 and 2 describes them as under the influence of deceiving demons to whom they open themselves up and give heed. That is not to say that all vegan leaders are apostates, but the strong spirits of deception and hypocrisy seem to operate through many of them, Christian and non-Christian alike, according to many testimonies of those closely involved.

We tend to notice these leaders deceiving others; however, first and foremost, they themselves are deceived. Earlier in this chapter you read of the incredible deception of T. C. Fry, another highly revered, national vegan leader. When he was dying of grave issues associated with his diet, he continued not only to deceive students, but tenaciously clung to that which was killing *him*. Living in total denial, he himself was first and foremost deceived beyond reality. That is an effect of being under the control of deceiving, lying spirits.

From the plethora of evidence, it seems that often one of several things happens to famous vegan leaders: 1) If they eat vegan long term, they develop serious health problems; then confess, change their diets, and are restored; or 2) if they continue on the diet, their health fails, and they may die; or 3) according to Gandhi, if they are in good health long term claiming to be vegans, they are frauds ("cheating," as some vegans refer to secretly eating animal-based foods). Few people are able to do well for the long term as vegetarians, certainly not as vegans I have known or known of.

Concerning the first of these, there are other vegan leaders who, like Nazariah, see the deterioration in their health from veganism, do not deny it when it surfaces. They humbly admit their mistake, apply the "brakes," and turn around before it is too late to help themselves and others they persuaded to join them in eating vegan. Another good example follows.

The Westbrooks Awaken In Time

Greg and Judie thought they "had it all," at first. "A Christian health ministry," perfect, personal health, and monetary rewards. What allurements! "How can it be wrong when it feels so right?" the song asks. They discovered the very disturbing truth.

Very strict vegans who followed the plan religiously, the Westbrook family found that six years into veganism, they sadly had to admit to themselves that they were no longer going forward. Rather they were seriously losing ground health wise, as were some others who had started the diet under Westbrooks' teaching. Greg reportedly lost a very large percentage of muscle and five teeth. In his thirties, he walked humped over. His wife, Judie, suffered excruciating, disabling headaches. The children were lethargic and chronically depressed; activities were no longer of interest to them.

"The more foods one eliminates from his/her diet, the greater the risk for nutritional deficiency," is a vital truth the family learned, before abandoning the vegan diet for God's whole menu.

After this family's dietary "trials of deficiencies," they wondered how many others were experiencing similar health problems. They took a vegan survey of symptoms for long-term dieters, and discovered to their astonishment, that the majority of the returned surveys listed numerous symptoms of deficiencies.[1] These were perhaps mostly Christian vegans who too had kept their issues quiet.

"Everyone I know on the [vegan] diet, is either "tinkering" with it, or under a doctor's care," Greg disclosed. He now alerts others, "If you've experienced new and troubling symptoms in your health, take heart. You haven't failed the [vegan] diet. The diet has probably failed you."[2]

"Be Fruitful & Multiply"

Thus our Creator instructed us, and gave us the diet important for procreating. Who, more than Christians, should have large families? God commanded it in order to provide Him godly offspring.[3] Yet Christian couples consuming a vegan diet may run into serious difficulties with pregnancies. The Foote's story that follows, is but one of a number of similar ones of which we are aware.

Andrew Foote and his wife, Romsey, visited a friend who experienced a "remarkable recovery from Lupus" with a popular Christian, vegan diet. They decided to learn more about it at a three day seminar with the leader and founder of the diet, who reportedly claimed the diet cured his tumor. While attending the training, they were amazed to learn of "so many others who had similar results of recovery from various health challenges after adopting this diet…" They also were taught to eliminate what was termed as the five

---

[1] itsyourhealth2.com/pages/testimony/deficiencies.htm
[2] Westbrook G, *When Hallelujah Becomes "What Happened!"* chetday.com/hallelujahwhathappenedreview
[3] Mal. 2:15. In the US, Muslims and Mexicans are producing a much higher percentage of births than Christians.

food "killers," i.e., meat, dairy, refined sugar, salt,[1] and refined white flour products. (Note the order and mixture of God's foods with the world's; and that meat and dairy quality vary.)

The Footes were completely convinced by what they heard at the training session, decided to "implement this diet 100%." Christians, they not only consumed it religiously. but also taught it for the next several years, thinking they had "found God's "ideal diet" based on His original eating instructions to man in Genesis 1:29," as the New Age church taught as well.

It was not until four years later, at a leaders' reunion, that they learned of the diet's deficiency in vitamin B_{12}. They were to obtain this with an occasional supplement and probiotics (intestinal flora). "We were convinced that to reintroduce meat back into our diet [in order to obtain vitamin B_{12}] was to reintroduce the number one food 'killer,'" Andrew said.

About six months later Romsey became pregnant. Her blood iron was low, but vitamin B_{12} level was normal. They "concluded with even stronger convictions..." that this "...was indeed God's 'ideal diet.'" (Studies show that blood test results for vitamin B_{12} are unreliable.) They were very careful not to "cheat," following the diet explicitly, Andrew says.

Several months after the baby was born, the Footes began noticing symptoms that concerned them. After nine months of breast feeding, the baby's muscle strength and motor skills were severely underdeveloped for his age. He could not crawl or hold his head up. Urine testing revealed vitamin B_{12} deficiency. Supplementation of the vitamin soon produced results; the baby was holding his head up within a few weeks and scooting around on his belly on the floor. However, when the first tooth came in at one year, it had no enamel. The parents added goat milk and subsequent teeth "came through" with enamel complete.

Vitamin B_{12}, calcium, iron – what else may be lacking in God's "ideal diet" this family wondered. Andrew lost a great deal of muscle due to protein deficiency. People noticed his slumping, and the Footes also lost a lot of weight before animal-source foods were added back to their diets.

---

[1] Sea salt is now allowed on the diet.

"In some ways, we feel duped," Andrew lamented. For the rest of the story, be sure to read Andrew's fascinating account online.[1]

God-Ordained Cooking

Some vegans eat a raw diet, some eat mostly raw. Scripture does not tell us that the Edenic diet was entirely raw. Nor does the New Testament, in instructing new believers, tell them to become vegetarians of any sort, but rather to eat meat that has been bled properly.[2]

It is not an essential though we think it is likely, that the Father taught Adam and Eve to eat cooked meat just before they left Eden. Their sons, Cain and Abel used fire for cooking meat and vegetables.

It is healthy to eat a good portion of our diet raw to prevent destruction of certain nutrients and enzymes by heat. Some people cannot tolerate a high amount of raw foods. Meat, grains, bread, beans and lentils, plus some other foods, are to be cooked, the Bible tells us. Recall that the Creator and Son of God, served the disciples fish He cooked over a fire. Sometimes meat was boiled.[3] Further, God told the Israelites *not* to eat the Passover lamb raw, but to roast it.[4]

Interestingly, a UK study of the effect of cooking and the digestibility of meat, found that

> ...Raw meat is seen to be far less readily digested *in vitro* than roast meat. **The maximum rate of digestion was obtained when meat was roasted so that when cut after cooling, it appeared a bright red color with a juicy surface.*** [Perhaps rare to medium rare.] Overcooking [well done] till the cold joint on cutting, appeared brown and dry, (though quite edible), markedly slowed the digestive rate, and this slowing occurred to an

---

[1] itsyourhealth2.com/pages/testimony/deficiencies.htm
[2] Acts 15:28, 29
[3] Lev. 8:31, Ezek. 46:20
[4] Ex. 12:8, 9

equal extent whether the application of heat were continuous or conducted in two successive periods [i.e., roasted, then leftovers reheated].[1]

*"This point probably coincides with that at which the anti-enzymic properties of animal tissues are destroyed, whilst the hardening and drying effect of heat on proteins has hardly come into play...Over-cooked meat is very slowly digested as compared with underdone meat...Re-warming underdone meat does not diminish its digestive rate of digestion," so long as it is only warmed.

In the wilderness, when the Israelites ate only that which Jehovah *Jirah* provided supernaturally, His chosen people cooked manna in various ways daily, except on Sabbath.

Some foods should always be cooked, though certainly in a healthy manner. Raw brassicas/cruciferous foods which suppress thyroid, e.g., kale, collards, cabbage, and broccoli, should be lightly steamed, not boiled. And of course, beans and grains should be soaked 24 hours, then simmered. The bioavailability of lycopene in tomatoes is increased with cooking. This phytonutrient improves cell communication's defense against cancer. Some people cannot tolerate a high raw foods.

Deep frying, bar-b-cue, ultrapasteurizing, and overcooking food, go way beyond the heat labile state (destroying or altering by heat). The highest level of leucocytosis (immune system reaction) is produced with the reactionary chemical configurations of such food preparation, without digestive enzymes to handle them well.

Studies show broccoli and Brussels sprouts are preventatives of colon cancer. They may act by increasing urinary excretion of potentially cancer-causing substances in well-done meat.[2] These foods should be lightly steamed or stir-fried, not eaten raw.

---

[1] Clifford MC, The effect of cooking on the digestibility of meat, Physiological Lab, King's Coll of Household & Soc Sci, Kensington, London, W 8, CXCII, Rec'd Oct. 23, 1930

[2] Hsu-LeBlanc E, Eat to beat cancer, *Natural Solutions*, Mar. 2007

Phony "Phoods"

At Christmas 2006, we received a beautiful vegetarian foods catalog in the mail. The front cover displayed a photo of the season's decorations, and a dining table laden with a Christmas meal. Pine boughs were in the background and were part of the centerpiece of large red apples stacked high, with red candles and walnuts on either side.

It was all displayed beautifully to appear to be a turkey dinner with all the trimmings, including a large pumpkin pie in the foreground. But upon looking more closely, we noticed that instead of a turkey, the main dish was a huge round squash with the top cut away, and filled with something unidentifiable. In front of it, what appeared to be a roast or meat dish of some kind, surrounded by vegetables, was actually an oblong, 2" high loaf of bread. Other dishes were pear halves with red cherries and green leaves in the centers; nuts, chocolate chip cookies, a dish of light colored vegetable, a goblet full of red berries, a tall wine bottle attractively tied with red serpentine ribbon and holly leaves, and nearby wine glasses filled with red wine. Beauty and the beast? Not!

While these may be mostly healthy foods, there was no meaningful source of protein, certainly no quality protein, and no fats to be seen on the table. Probably the fat in the cookies was margarine. The foods were all entirely all sources of high carbs. How disappointing. It appeared to promise much, but nothing there that would "stick to the ribs," provide satiety, or serious nutrition. *Au contraire.* The top of the page simply read *Holiday 2006*.

Most vegan diets, being very restrictive, become creative with recipes referring to foods by names which have no resemblance to what they actually are, e.g., the "raw 'cereal" has not a trace of cereal in it. Counterfeit "milk" (soy, almond, rice, *et al*) in no way resembles the nutrient-dense real milk provided by our Creator, as mentioned numerous times in the Bible; soy "bacon" has no pork, tofu "turkey" has no turkey. Why do vegetarians/vegans call their foods by names that sound like animal-based ones they so detest? It would seem they would not wish them to sound *anything* like that which they avoid like the plague!

Shortening Lives – God's Purpose For Meat?

One group of Christian vegans teaches that God purposely "allowed" fallen, sinful man's flesh-eating, in order to shorten his life span. Allow me to give you some food for thought about this outrageous proposal!.

Did Jesus feed fish to his chosen apostles to shorten their lives, knowing they would require nutrient-dense foods to enable them to carry out His Great Commission to evangelize the world? Would Peter have hurriedly jumped out of the boat to get to Jesus on the shore, if he had known the One he trusted with his life, was actually cooking something He knew would shorten it?

God himself ate meat, milk and butter with Abraham.[1] Yet if it is His will to shorten man's life through meat-eating, would He not have told His trusting friend to eat it *three times daily or more*? And would His Word lovingly teach us moderation, warning us to "Eat only so much as is *good* for thee"? If He wants us to die sooner, He has complete control of that. Our days are in His hands.

The book of Leviticus alone, and a great deal else in the Bible, teaches man how to *avoid* an early death, and which meats to eat. If an early death is God's plan, why not eat any and everything?

In fact, Moses declared we are to honor parents in order that our days may be *long* on the earth. This law giver also instructed God's people in eating meat. Is the Fifth Commandment promise to vegetarians only?

Psalm 107:38 declares God's blessing upon His people's lives, not shortening of them. How can one consider the following passage from Deuteronomy 7:11, 13-15 which includes the Creator's blessing on food animals, and yet believe that God intended or allowed meat in order to shorten man's life span through disease? Not only did He *not* do that with fresh, animal-based foods, but they are a special, nourishing gift from Him as we have shown. Meat animals are referred to here by God as part of His *abundant* blessing, associated not with shortened lives, but with wellness.

---

[1] Obviously milk was not intended for babies only, as some teach. Prov. 27:27, 1 Cor. 9:7

11. Thou shalt therefore keep the commandments, the statutes, and the judgments which I command thee this day, to do them...

13. And He will love thee, and **bless** thee, and **multiply** thee: He will **also bless** the fruit of thy womb, and the fruit of thy land, thy corn and thy wine, and thine oil, **the increase of thy kine [cattle], and the flocks of thy sheep...**

14. Thou shalt be **blessed** above all people: there shall not be male or female barren among you, **or among your cattle**.

15. And the Lord will take away from thee all sickness, and will put none of the evil diseases of Egypt [the world], which thou knowest, upon thee, but will lay them upon all them that hate thee.

Here we are specifically told that obedience brings fertility and God's blessing on man, *and* on his animal-based and other food; that it is the breaking of God's law ("Sin is the transgression of the law."), including His dietary law of eating green vegetables with meat, as well as modern unhealthy food preparation, which lead to sickness and death. Could the blessing of man and his food, bring a shortened life? Was God's blessing actually wrapped in a curse?

Would there not be a credibility issue in trusting God and anything He instructs us to do in His Word, if it were true that meat itself shortens lives? Such false teaching seems to us "The foolishness of man [which] perverts his way, and his heart frets against God," declares Proverbs 19:3.

Compounded costs of man's incredibly destructive disobedience from Eden forward, account for the shortened life span. To even suggest that he no longer lives to Methusela's 969 years because the Father knowingly provided meat to drastically reduce man's longevity, is worse than wicked, it seems to me.

It was not necessary for God to stoop to nefarious, underhanded schemes to reduce man's life span, if that were His aim. Rather our good God *intervened* to maintain it as high as 70-

80 years for this long![1] My Father instructed me to eat meat, therefore meat is good for me.

In Genesis 1:28, 29, we read:

> And God blessed them [Adam and Eve] and said unto them: "Be fruitful, and multiply, and replenish the earth, and subdue it: have dominion over the fish of the sea, and over the fowl of the air, and over every living thing that moves upon the earth."
>
> And God said, "Behold, I have given you every herb bearing seed, which is upon the face of all the earth, and every tree, in the which is the fruit of a tree yielding seed; to you it shall be for meat [Heb. *ok-law*, food or meat].

Later, when Noah and his family came out of the ark, in Genesis 9 we learn that

> ...God blessed Noah and his sons, and said unto them, "Be fruitful, and multiply and replenish the earth. And the fear of you and the dread of you shall be upon every beast of the earth, and upon every fowl of the air, upon all that **moves** upon the earth, and upon all the fishes of the sea; into your hand are they delivered. Every **moving** thing that lives shall be meat [same Hebrew word as in Genesis 1:29, *ok-law*] for you; even as the green herb have I given you all things. But flesh with the life thereof, which is the blood thereof, shall ye not eat..."[2]

In Genesis 9, man no longer had dominion over submissive animals necessary for loading and containing them on the ark; instead came fear of him, with animals added as part of man's diet.

There were other reasons animals would became useful to man (work, clothing, milk products) but here God specifically commands man regarding "...moving animals which shall be meat for you..."

---

[1] Psa. 90:10

[2] This is the same Word the Jerusalem church leaders gave new believers: "Eat meat, be sure it's bled properly."

The wisdom of man puts two and two together, and comes up with something like this: "The GI track is too long to process meat; it was designed to process only raw fruits and vegetables with fiber; since flesh food has no fiber, it sits in the bowel and putrefies, whether raised organically or not, or properly prepared. And this putrefaction causes colon cancer and many other very bad diseases."

First, that's bad science, both with respect to anatomy, and as regards poor, outdated studies of fiber and it's effectiveness against cancer. Second, we must ask why these modern day diseases did not manifest during the many thousands of years since man began eating meat.

Also note that it's not just corrupted meat produced from foods unnatural for livestock consumption, plus grained animals given antibiotics, growth hormones, treated with pesticides and other toxins; plus human consumption of countless factory foods with trans fats, rancid oils, and myriad toxins of their own, that sit in the colon due to constipation and other lack of peristalsis.

Should we hold God responsible for all these diseases, who after all, told man to eat meat, knowing full well man's large intestine was "designed only for fibrous plant foods," that meat has no fiber, would just sit there and rot, and that man would develop a host of horribly painful diseases as a result of the toxicity from eating meat as he was told to do? That is exactly what some vegan Christians today are accusing God of doing for the purpose of reducing the life span of wicked man, they speculate.

All good, earthly parents try to prevent their children from eating that which is not good for them. Would our loving Father even suggest, much less command us, to eat that which He knew would cause us to become diseased, suffer horribly, and die early?

Would God expect man to multiply and replenish the earth if meat would make him so ill? The answer is no to both these questions! The Creator knew man would fall and gave him an omnivorous digestive system in the beginning, that would process both plant and flesh foods.

Repeatedly in Genesis 9, and before that in the sixth chapter of the same book, God tells Noah He will establish His covenant with this righteous believer. A covenant in those days was a completely binding agreement, requiring the death of anyone who broke it.

One did not enter into a covenant with those whose word could not be trusted to the death.

Noah completely trusted God, and obeyed under extremely trying conditions for 120 years while he preached to the totally corrupt and violent inhabitants, even giants, and built the unique ark. Clearly Noah believed God was a good God, of the utmost integrity, and who wanted only his children's best. There is no record that he ever questioned this.

Unlike today's educated vegan leaders, for certain, it never occurred to Noah to wonder if his God would deceptively "bless" his children with a gift that would cause many debilitating diseases, including everything from colon cancer to Crohn's disease, as some vegan leaders lists them.

Is this a subtle teaching questioning the loving character of God Almighty, or His lack of knowledge of all things beforehand and since the Fall, or is it a false doctrine based upon a profound lack of knowledge of both Scripture and science?

The Bible assures us that every gift from above is good and perfect for that which He intends it.[1] Has it not been only since the advent of fabricated foods (replacing God's organic, fresh, whole ones), chronic stress and chronic toxic emotions; chlorinated[2] and polluted water, and man's environmental toxins, that all the GI track diseases incorrectly being associated with fresh, clean meat, have come to be?

Shortly we will address fiber's importance, or lack of it. Remember, that after a year of thriving on *nothing but meat for a year,* Dr. Stefansson was declared healthy by the world's most respected medical authorities!

Woe Unto Them That Call Good Bad...[3]

One vegan diet's cornbread recipe states that "**eggs,** shortening, and sugar are all bad ingredients." The recipes do not differentiate between the world's destructive foods (we know who

---

[1] James 1:16, 17
[2] Chlorinated water kills both bad and good bacteria (probiotics, the very valuable friendly bacteria).
[3] Isa. 5:20

is the ruler of this world[1]) and the Creator's healthy, restorative ones. God did not create highly processed foods.

Wrote Ellen G. White, prophetess of the Seventh Day Adventists: "We bare positive testimony against tobacco, rich cakes, spiritous liquors, snuff, tea, coffee, **flesh meats, butter,** spice, mince pies."[2]

To us it seems nothing short of sacrilege to lump devitalized, stripped, non-foods, liquor, and tobacco together with God's nutrient-dense foods. This same lack of distinguishing between real and counterfeit foods – between foods that nurture and restore, and foods that lead to disease and death - is found in the conventional nutrition community of the world.

A secular handout for patients being tested for CVD and osteoporosis, advises "a no-nonsense approach" that supposedly will lower the risk of a host of serious diseases, including these. Of course the first way to do this, it was explained, is by being certain to lower cholesterol levels (whatever they may be).

So what was the supposed most effective way to do this? Of course, "by avoiding saturated and transfats." How? By limiting the use of butter, margarine, and shortening. Patients were also advised to avoid red meat, eggs, fried foods, commercially packaged cakes and cookies, doughnuts, and French fries. What a mixture of information and *mis*information! One might conclude all these sources "march to the same drummer." It is disturbing when Christians parrot conventional nutritional wisdom of this caliber.

In the order of importance, the Greeks listed the most important first. As also here. Did you notice that first in grouping of foods to avoid were red meats, eggs, and butter, dating back to the Prudent Diet, still alive and well today. How subtly America's masses are conditioned day after day by the world *and* Christian leaders, as *our Maker's real food is listed together and equated with the "bad" to be avoided.*

Again, in the secular educational handout, the value of meat was diminished as a source of "bad" fat. Soybeans, "…**thought** to be particularly heart healthy," plus legumes, are "all 'good'

---

[1] John 16:11
[2] Testimonies to the Church, Vol. 3, p. 21.

choices" as well, in addition to low-fat dairy, skinless chicken breasts, and egg whites or egg substitutes. (Note the reference here is not to soy but to soy*beans* coupled with "good" beans, peas and lentils. Who eats soy*beans?*

The superior whole egg nourishment is rejected due to fat in the yolk. Low-fat dairy, skinless chicken, egg whites only, or egg substitute - so many ways they pervert and devitalize the Creator's whole and wholesome foods![1]

Did divine wisdom not include fat in milk, skin on chicken, and yolks (yes, with fat!) in eggs? Then why is the wisdom of the world considered superior by so many of God's people who "swallow it hook, line, and sinker"? In spite of years of the low fat diet, CVD is still the number one cause of death by disease.[2]

Is It All About Fiber?

The front cover of the book, *Fiber Menace,* pictures a large cereal bowl filled with metal, threaded, sharp screws. You wouldn't dream of eating such for breakfast or any other time! Konstantin Monastyrsky, the author, a former vegetarian, tells of his near-death experience after years of the modern diet craze low in fats and protein, and high in fiber.[3] This certified nutritionist and former pharmacologist (researcher of the interaction of drugs and chemicals with biological systems), found that eating a high fiber diet with large amounts of grains, fruits, vegetables, and legumes, actually leads to some of the worst intestinal diseases they are touted to prevent.

Monastyrsky explains that our digestive systems were designed chiefly for protein digestion, with small amounts of fiber. Protein residue is digested in individuals with normal digestion (most of the stool should be bacteria), does not sit in the colon. If we consume excess fiber, digestion is slowed, fermentation occurs, threatening flora, causing bloating, gas, large stools, constipation

---

[1] The sources of all this misinformation were reported as some of America's elitist health organizations and medical schools, as parroed by all today.

[2] See also Death By Medicine, Null, G, Dean, C, Feldman, M, Rasio, D, & Smith, D, *Life Extension* magazine and online, Aug. 2006-67-87, indepth report of scientific studies of iatrogenic related deaths in the US.

[3] Ageless Press; ffibermenace.com, as viwed May 2006

or diarrhea, Irritable Bowel Syndrome, and diverticular disease. As a result, trauma is inflicted upon the gastrointestinal mucosa by the expansion of the fiber, this scientist explains.

Supported by myriad medical studies, *Fiber Menace* emphasizes that a high fiber diet is not only unhealthy, it is unnecessary for bowel movements.[1] In fact, according to Harvard School of Public Health, earlier studies were largely based on "a broad look at large groups of people." Some case control studies (memory reliance) showed fiber was linked to lower risk of colon cancer, but many others did not. It was not until cohort studies of groups of people were performed over a period of time, and bolstered by randomized study results, that it became clear that "fiber intake had very little, if any, link with colon cancer." If scientist Monastyrsky's findings are anywhere near accurate, it may be on the contrary; high fiber intake may *contribute* to colon disease.

The American College of Gastroenterology Functional Gastrointestinal Disorders Task Force, found that "none of the legitimate clinical trials demonstrated that fiber causes 'improvement in stool frequency or consistency when compared with placebo.'

Yet a chief reason most vegans (Christian and non-Christian) believe meat is bad is its lack of fiber.[2] According to that theory, eating a great deal of fiber (or taking fiber products) is important for healthy bowel function. (Some fiber is important, though not for the reason most believe; we will address this shortly.)

If fiber is an essential for moving meat residue through the body, wouldn't God have commanded Noah and the rest of us, to eat lots and lots of it along with the meat? On the other hand, if He wanted to shorten our lives, and the present theory is true, would He have told Noah to eat greens?

---

[1] The author warns against suddenly reducing fiber. See that book for "how to."
[2] Biochemically, fiber is a non-starch, unavailable polysaccharide subclass of complex carbohydrates, with major components of lignin (makes vegetables firm), pectins (apple), cellulose (wood pulp), and mucilage (okra). It does not break down into simple sugars during passage through the GI tract on the way to excretion in the stool. Fiber is present chiefly in the cell walls of plant foods.

Supported by "scores of studies," Monastyrsky found that too much fiber over expands the colon, and *increases* constipation and the risk for colon disease.[1] However, it can be said that but for trying to eat a high fiber diet, many people would eat only "factory foods."

Remember we discussed conjugated lenoleic acid (CLA), an *un*saturated fatty acid found only in red meat, whole milk, and whole milk derivatives, that provides powerful properties that actually inhibit colorectal cancer (CRC). But further on in this section we will show that amazing as CLA is, the Creator didn't stop there in providing prevention for this disease.

The fiber thing seems to have begun with Kellogg before the forties, and later with the breakfast cereal of the PD.[2] In 1969, Burkitt's hypothesis[3] first proposed that dietary fiber was protective against CRC, diverticulitis, and other gastrointestinal diseases. Several studies showed an inverse association between dietary fiber and reduced incidents of CRC. However, about half dozen superior, recent studies[4] and clinical trials, including the Nurses Health Study, reported "no relation between fibre intake and colon cancer incidence;...increased dietary fibre intake did not reduce colorectal adenoma recurrence..."[5] Nor was there any decrease in all-cause mortality; in fact, high fiber intake in a large study of post-myocardial infarction men, "...if anything, showed that mortality was higher" with those increasing dietary fiber intake. Nearly 60 years after the onset of the PD, finally sanity: "High fiber cereals may not be that good for you after all," was the *International Journal of Epidemiology* conclusion.

The Good Guys

A chief benefit of a small amount of fermentable fiber, is not to keep meat moving (healthy digestion takes care of that residue);

---

[1] http://www.fibermenace.com/Fiber-Menace-Intro.pdf
[2] http://www.fibermenace.com/Fiber-Menace-Intro.pdf , as viewed June 2007
[3] Burkitt DP, Related Disease-Related Cause, *Lancet,* 1969, 1971
[4] See Chapter Three regarding differences in the kinds of studies.
[5] Mai V, *et al*, Dietary fibre and risk of colorectal cancer in the Breast Cancer Detection Demonstration Project (BCDDP) follow-up cohort, *Int Jnl of Epidemiology,*2003;32:234-239

but for feeding colon flora, "the good guys." In fact, the bowel is part of a most complex ecosystem that is populated by a multitude of living organisms interacting with one another and us, their hosts. These microbes are always eating, and eliminating their own wastes. They are extremely involved with our health or disease; for better or for worse, depending upon whether the friendly or unfriendly microorganisms are in control of the territory. Yet most people have never heard of intestinal flora.

Some of these microorganisms (probiotics) contribute only to our health. For example, they manufacture vitamin B, produce lactase enzyme for digesting dairy foods; are anti-carcinogenic (anti-cancer); have powerful potential as anti-tumor factors; prevent spreading of the disease-causing microbes; enhance our immune systems, **peristalsis and bowel function to prevent constipation, toxification, and disease;** and promote a healthy intestinal lining. A high percentage of acne may be controlled by these. Intestinal flora even help to lower cholesterol. Indeed, a long list of conditions has been shown to respond to healthy levels of good intestinal bacteria: cystitis, colitis and many other bowel problems, psoriasis, eczema, arthritis, gout, and cancer.

Abnormal microorganisms can make us ill or even kill us (overgrowth of fungi, yeasts, viruses, bacteria) if a balance is not maintained. It is not an exaggeration to say that our lives depend upon the three and one-half pounds of the 400 strains of friendly bacteria in our digestive tracts (approximately one-third of the dry weight of fecal material is bacteria), and whether or not we see to it that they have a healthy environment in which to work and reproduce.[1]

Poor diet, chronic stress, and toxins are hard on the "good guys." Chlorine and some other chemicals, as well as broad spectrum antibiotics, are not selective in the kinds of bacteria they destroy. If good bacteria are not replaced in the gut, and pathogenic (disease producing) microorganism numbers proliferate excessively, so will the toxic by-products of the latter, increasingly

---

[1] Approximately 60% of full term babies born vaginally are found to have colonized flora, compared with only 9% of Caesarean section births. Probiotics are vital for getting infants off to a good start digestively.

and adversely affecting the lining of the bowel and intestines. Over time, digestion, and absorption also suffer.

Some physicians recommend daily intakes of viable yogurt,[1] probiotic supplementation, or sauerkraut, to help overcome this deficiency (dysbiosis) after a course of antibiotics, or in cases of Irritable Bowel Syndrome (IBS), with which approximately 20% of Americans suffer. Viable yogurt cultures also predigest protein, and enhance that digestion and absorption for so many with less than optimum digestion.

Remember the greens God commanded Noah to eat with the meat? It's not only their fiber, but today we also know that *Lactobacillus plantarum*, is found on raw green vegetable leaves. This strain may be the most beneficial microorganism for maintaining healthy bowels. With each bite of obedience, Noah maintained his. So should we.

The Biblical ancients also consumed daily amounts of cultured raw milk products such as sour milk, yogurt, and real kefir (not to be confused with the sugary drinks sold today by that name), supplying good bacteria for many good reasons. The good bacteria "thrive on fat,"[2] the bad ones on simple sugars.

"...[U]nfermented grains contain chemicals that irritate and inflame the bowel wall, and can even cause it to spasm. The practice of consuming large amounts of [unsoaked] whole grains and rough bran, which has been the cornerstone of treatment for constipation, can actually lead to IBS," advises Dr. Cowan.[3] Remember Susan Seimer's testimony? "Since giving up my vegetarian ways in late 2000, my hypoglycemia is virtually symptomless, my bowels are working right again," she testified.

Do Vegans Really Live Longer?

The largest study of "true mortality rates of vegetarians and vegans" was published a few years ago, demonstrating that though

---

[1] We have found very few commercial yogurt products to have viable probiotic cultures at time of purchase. We enjoy homemade plain yogurt with stevia. Avoid those with sugary fruit and such.

[2] Cowan T, Ask The Doctor About Irritable Bowel Syndrome, *Wise Traditions,* Weston A. Price Foundation

[3] *Ibid.*

we all have been led to believe that vegans live longer, their life span is actually shorter than other dietary groups. According to Nazariah, who agonized over the study results published in the vegan magazine, *Ahimsa,*[1] showed that vegans suffer a higher rate of degenerative brain diseases, including Alzheimer's, dementia, and others. The vegan diet does not adequately support the central nervous system (CNS).

Furthermore, all the positive stats about vegans, that "they suffer less this and that,"including the many benefits of that diet as put forth in the media, books, and at artful websites, were not derived from large people groups who died, explained Nazariah candidly in his interview with Padenaude. It was all merely extrapolated info, not actual. In other words, it was estimated by projecting known information. However, it turns out that the "known information" may not have been factual.

For example, most Americans and many others today still believe that fats cause cardiovascular disease. Since vegans are said to eat 30% less fat,[2] ergo, they will suffer 30% less heart disease, as the statistics are quoted. The problem with that hypothesis is that the superior studies show that fat does *not* cause CVD. Therefore the conclusion cannot be true. Even if fat were the culprit, it does not necessarily follow that 30% less fat would ensure 30% less heart disease since there are other causative factors involved with that issue.

Another one is chronic stress, including stress deriving from nutritional deficiencies, which is high for most all in this day and age, regardless of best diets. The flawed statistic published in respect to vegans and CVD, is but one of the many Nazariah has found to be all theory.

It's not as if this former vegan came by his present position overnight. He explained that he had done due diligence in his research of many studies, and had discussions with many expert practitioners with extensive clinical experience with vegans.

---

[1] Visit the fascinating Ahimsa website at Ahimsa.com. Utterly amazing what you'll find!

[2] From my professional experience and what I observe in a local vegetarian deli, I question that figure. Vegans avoid saturated fat to a great extent, however, they may consume other fats in large amounts.

There was also a longevity study of women published in the 1990s in the *Vegetarian Times* magazine, well known to vegans. Of the three groups – meat eaters, lacto-ovo vegetarians, and vegans, L-O vegetarians lived the longest, meat eaters second, and vegans have the *shortest* life spans. (Unless indicated, such studies are not done with organic meat as stated earlier in this book. Non-organic meats often have nitrates, hormones, antibiotics, are irradiated, and may have other unhealthy conditions. Neither do we know what else the meat eaters consumed, their lifestyles, etc. Even so, in this study, veganism placed last.)

Though vegans may aspire to 120 years of age, I have never met one vegan centenarian. Have you? I have known a few older than 100 who were not vegetarians. Genes, toxic environment; severe, chronic stress; "eating at the world's table,"[1] or things we have no control over - all may impact health and how long we will live this side of Eden.

Psalm 90:10 tells us that God allotted the "number of our days" to 70 years; and depending upon one's strength, one might live to 80. This range is where fallen man generally "leveled off." No one will die prematurely in the Millennium, even then "the child shall die a hundred years old," not 120. [2]

It is true we *can* make a dramatic difference in the *quality* of our lives and greatly reduce sickness events, so that we are more available for good works. *That* has been my aim, not to live to 120 years of age or anything near that. The desire to be with our Lord, and the mind boggling, increasing wickedness of this world, have created a longing for heaven.

We may certainly avoid a great deal of prolonged and needless suffering physiologically, by eating the Creator's fresh whole foods, choosing a healthy life- style, exercising, getting adequate rest, and being right with God and our fellow man. Yet we cannot expect on average, to live more than our allotted days. The 70-80 years of Scripture is not a promise but a principle.

There are few exceptions anymore. A relative died at 112 years of age, but his daughter lived about 40 years fewer. My

---

[1] The one who "writes the menus" for the world's table, came to kill, steal, and destroy.
[2] Isa. 65:20

mother is in her nineties. But those genes, formed when fresh whole foods with significantly more nutrients than today, are fast fading. It will be only by following God's plan for eating after the Fall, that succeeding generations will live to be 70 or 80 years of age, and enjoy good quality of life, if the world lasts.

The Whole Counsel of God...

Even if it were possible to obtain the Genesis 1:29 diet today, if we could eat even a fraction of *every* kind of seed-bearing, green plant and fruit, it would not be adequate for our bodies. We must not stop with one verse of the Bible given to perfect people. We absolutely must consider and obey the *whole* Word. From early childhood we learned 2 Timothy 2:15 teaching us to "study to show [ourselves] approved unto God, a workman that needs not to be ashamed, rightly dividing the Word of truth." Again, text without context equals pretext. Here the context is the *whole* Word of God, not just forty-one words from one verse on page one! No one can question that animal-based foods are found throughout Scripture, were eaten by God's chosen people, and God himself according to His Word.

In Romans 14 we have two exceptions. There Paul refers to a brother who is ignorant of Bible teaching as to his liberty (is weak in the faith), and believes he should not eat meat offered to the idols he used to worship. The other exception is that we are not to unnecessarily offend such a brother (eat meat before him). To walk in faith and love is most important, the apostle was teaching there.

Healing & Veganism

"But I have a friend who was suffering a serious health condition; he went on a vegan diet, and got well," you may respond. So how *are* those impressive healings explained? It's not as complicated as one may think.

Today's vegan converts were often taking multiple toxic drugs.[1] As well, they were usually acidic and toxic from

---

[1] Recent news reports avg. American takes 12 prescription drugs each year, to say nothing of over the counter ones - most all toxic.

constipation and fabricated-foods' unnatural ingredients and additives. They were consuming large amounts of highly processed vegetable oils (usually soy) and trans fats. They drank little water but gallons of sodas. The liver and kidneys were sluggish and doing poor jobs detoxifying it all.

With an all raw vegan diet they stop consuming white bread, pasta, pie, cake, cookies, candy, chips, ultrapasteurized milk, cured meats with nitrites, processed cheeses, sugary cereals, shakes, and soda drinks, and other refined carbs; coffee, fried chicken, French fries, hot dogs, transfats, and highly processed polyunsaturates. (Cancer thrives on sugar, and in the acidic environment created by non-foods.)

Feeling better, they may begin exercising, getting more sunshine, and drinking more water. And their physicians may take them off toxic drugs the physicians deem no longer necessary.

After years of the Standard American Diet (SAD), and with a new diet of more easily digested and assimilated real food, including large amounts of *whole* foods, often it does not take long to experience even dramatic improvement. Think about it…is it surprising if we stop taking in many of the various toxins into our bodies, remove the ones already there, and then provide drastically improved nutrition (most anything would be better!), that our bodies would begin the healing work they are designed to do?

In fact, this is exactly the way the Creator designed them to begin rejuvenation. Scripture tells us His fresh good foods renew our youth like eagles who have been through a fasting molt![1]

Raw juices, fruits and vegetables, are mostly alkaline and cleansing. They help balance the body's pH. The overburdened eliminating organs - liver, kidneys, bowels, skin, and lungs, are relieved when the heavy toxin load is significantly reduced. The "trash" in the blood is carried out, and it begins purification. The previous toxic river to the liver and kidneys, and the rest of the body, eases, depending upon whether organic foods are eaten.[2]

---

[1] Psa. 103:5; 107:38.

[2] Besides chemical toxicity, the typical non-organic crop receives 10 applications of estrogen-type, endocrine-disrupting chemicals, "from seed to storage." Klein L, Why Farmers Use Hormones, WAPF for *Wise Traditions*

Digestion and metabolism improve. How could the wellness level *not* improve with those drastic differences!

Again, when we stop or remove what is causing the problem, and provide the body more of what it needs nutritionally, including fluids from broths and fresh foods, it often heals itself. Most often it isn't too late for marked degree of it. The body luxuriates in the dietary intake of real food.

Though the nutrition is limited, the restoration may slowly and gradually continue for years, depending upon the individual and the choice of foods. For the short haul, thrilled with an almost certain new level of wellness, the new vegans believe they have reached "Nirvana."

They excitedly continue the diet for a period, lose weight, sleep better, have more energy for a time, and feel very good, or at least better. But eventually – and it varies for individuals – the body begins to tell them that something more is needed. We have previously mentioned the many signs of malnutrition, including neurological disorders and muscle and bone loss.

After The Summit...

Due to toxins in our environment, food, water, internal microbial emissions, metabolic[1] and other internal wastes mostly stored in fatty tissue, an annual cleansing and restoration for various numbers of weeks, is healthy for most. This leads to relative resting of the liver and digestive systems in particular. We were created with bodies that constantly work to achieve homeostasis;[2] when we remove that which hinders this, the body most often heals itself.

With veganism, and other very restrictive diets, the cleansing may continue for years. Long before that, profound detoxification is no longer needed or helpful. Indeed, it becomes detrimental, and the nutrition level insufficient.

I have observed that often when former, long-time vegans begin adding flesh foods to their diets, after short periods of only

---

[1] Metabolism is the sum of chemcial reactions in living cells..
[2] Homeostasis involves an organism's or cell's continued adjustment of its physiological processes to maintain equilibrium, including continual healing.

small amounts at meals, the level of wellness repeatedly plateaus until more meat is added, together with dairy products (raw, if available). The former vegan nurse I told you about earlier, is an example. The previously starving cells, organs, and systems come to life, and cry out for more nourishment to maintain their exciting new level, and won't settle for less! Though eating meat may still be repulsive to them, they begin to have increasing energy and feel noticeably better. Or like Linda, they may say, "It felt so right to my body!" When this happens, vegans should listen to their bodies, and provide them that for which they clamor.

Yet I have not seen in any other group, the extreme zeal of the adherents of veganism. They appear to focus upon the idea of a vegan diet, *per se*, to the exclusion of what their bodies may be screaming at them.

Like a B_{12} deficiency, it may take years to recognize in some cases, but sooner or later the need for more nutrition will manifest to trained practitioners even if not obvious to the patient who has learned to live with conditions. There's very good reason the body is no longer keeping up with demands placed upon it.

Like the remodeling of a house, we can remove only so much before we must begin putting major new materials back in. In the long term, "the human body is better able to cope with less cleansing than less nutrition," as a wise one observed. That is true for many diets that may work for some people for a time.

Let's be clear: though fruits and vegetables may contain important, needed nutrients and phytonutrients, they are not nutrient-dense foods required especially today. Some are almost nutritionally worthless, depending upon soil, transport, storage, and other devitalizing conditions. "Camping" as a vegan may be beneficial for a short time, but don't build your nutrition "house" there.

It is essential to consider all the evidence, the whole picture, the long term, when we talk about a vegetarian diet, and especially a vegan one. Never lose sight of that principle since the media and seemingly every other avenue of expression these days, keeps before the unknowing public the alleged risks of animal-based foods versus oft proclaimed health benefits of vegetarianism. We aren't getting the whole story and the sobering facts.

I am repeating this point because it is important to drive home. Because Aunt Susie recovered with a vegan diet, and the partial regimen served a purpose and was a vast improvement over the previous diet, does *not* mean it will be adequate indefinitely. After the body responds with its initial, significant improvement, it does all it can with the limited nutrients, then it may begin to lose momentum.

"The Brick Wall" They Are "Butting Their Heads" Against

After the Fall of mankind, and down through the millennia, myriad deficiencies have gradually increased. The last 20 years have seen a dramatic rate in loss of nutrients in plant foods. During the short period from 1975 through 1997, plant nutrients diminished significantly, according to USDA data. Just to name a few, average calcium levels in a dozen fresh vegetables were reduced 27%. Vitamin A dropped 21%; vitamin C a whopping 30%; and iron almost 40%!

Dr. Robert L. Lawrence wrote:

> Foods grown on [American] soils therefore lack the vital nutrients, processes and enzymes that were originally placed. The lack of these compounds ultimately leads to disease within the organism consuming them.[1]

Can vegetarians increase vitamin supplementation to overcome all this? I think not. Pasture soils are also losing nutrients, meaning meats are losing their levels of nutrition as well; all the more reason organic meats can be an increasing boost.

We cannot reasonably expect today's aging earth to produce pre-Fall quality foods, or even a small amount of that which the Israelites found when they spied out Canaan.[2] The latter's rich soil was so teeming with life that one bunch of grapes required two men to carry it supported by two poles resting on their shoulders!

---

[1] Lawrence, R., *From the Doctor's Office,* Garden Gazette, Feb. 2005
[2] Even so, our spinach leaves are approx. 15"x8", broccoli heads approx. 8" wide. Not too bad 7,000 yrs. after Eden.

Have you seen such in our day? No, and you won't before the new Millennium of Christ's rule and reign on a new earth.

What we have today is a tiny fraction of the nutritional resources available during those times, and studies show we are fast losing that. In no way does our food approach even post-Eden levels of nutrition, much less Eden's itself as in Genesis 1:29.

All the fruits and vegetables, supplements and adjuncts vegans consume, of whatsoever kind anywhere, cannot make up for the profound difference in nourishment, then and now (pre- and post-Fall). The depleted soils, pesticides, global transporting, processing, additives, storage, preservation, and final food preparations – all play serious parts in diminishing of nutrients, depending upon the quantity and quality initially. Far more is needed.

Every kind and most of America's foods, have been very seriously devitalized by many and varied practices. Yet no one is fighting eating fruits and vegetables, only animal-based foods. Neither dare we throw out all animal-based foods because most have been "abused" in this fallen world. As consumers are increasingly demanding them, there are more and more nearby and online organic, grass-fed cattle farms, usually family farms. We need to support them as much as possible!

Thankfully consuming the Creator's special animal-source food gifts can do wonders in making up for the monumental loss with the fall. It is not enough, yet it is critical. *Whatever* we do to enhance our nutrition, is 100% better than doing nothing, and can make a significant difference!

As the Father provided additional, compensatory nourishment after the Fall, so He has also in this end time when the need is exponentially greater. That is a chief theme of the 1 Timothy 4:1-6 passage.

Above All, Get Wisdom (Use "Common Sense"!)

Does it make any sense then that in the end time when nutrients are disappearing from the diet at an alarming rate, that God would have us eat none of the most nutrient-rich foods?

Countless good things such as American history, literature, music, and sex, now have been corrupted, even Bibles versions.

But we don't exclude all, rather we follow godly principles in our choices. We must do the same with animal-source foods.

It bears repeating that in Acts 15:20, the Jerusalem council didn't tell Gentile converts to eat vegetables only, or not to eat meat, but not to eat strangled animals, which had not been bled properly.[1] That's not a vegetarian Church.

FYI: Daniel's Choice

Some Christians cite the prophet Daniel as an example of a biblical vegan. "Here's God's plan for eating," they say regarding Daniel 1, "he ate the Genesis 1:29 diet." However, from chapter ten, verse three of that book, we know that the prophet did not remain on pulse (dried beans, seeds, grains) indefinitely. He specifically recorded that *while fasting* he ate no "pleasant bread or flesh," indicating that after the three weeks he returned to a diet including these.

Because the pagans ate a great deal of unclean foods prepared in unhealthy ways, likely Daniel ate pulse for the three year period of training until he was free to resume a greater variety of the full bounty of God's nutritional provision, including clean, animal-based foods, and fresh fruits and vegetables. It was not ceremonial defilement but pollution from Persian delicacies as the Hebrew has it, that caused Daniel to opt for the pulse. After Peters' vision in Acts 10, he did not argue about eating meat in general; it was eating *unclean* meat that bothered him.

It Was Prophesied

> 1. Now the Spirit speaks expressly, that in the latter times some shall depart **from the faith**, giving heed to seducing spirits, and doctrines of devils;
> 2. Speaking lies in hypocrisy; having their conscience seared with a hot iron;
> 3. ...commanding to abstain from meats which God has created to be received with thanksgiving of them which believe and know the truth.

---

[1] Gen. 9:4

4. For every creature of God is good, and nothing is to be refused if it is received with thanksgiving:
5. For it is sanctified by the Word of God and prayer.
6. If thou put the brethren in remembrance of these things, thou shalt be a good minister of Jesus Christ, nourished up in the words of faith and of good doctrine, whereunto thou has attained.[1]

Vegan/vegetarian diets are in direct conflict with, and disobedient to, this and other passages of the Word. This text couples abstaining from meat God created to be eaten, with departing from the faith. Rather than giving thanks for these special, God-given good gifts to be eaten from the Fall down through the millennia, and especially in the endtime in which we live, Christian vegetarian/vegan adherents strongly reject them, sometimes referring to them as "killer foods." This seems to us a "slap in the face" of our loving Father who provided nutrient-dense foods after Eden for their particular nourishment and unique properties. This becomes a spiritual matter as well as a health issue.

Missing Scriptures?

Nothing in the entire Bible instructs man to continue eating a vegan diet after the Fall. However, there *are* a number of commandments to eat animal-based foods, with many examples in both the Old and New Testaments.

As we saw, God teaches His people in Exodus 15:26, that if they will listen to His commandments and *do* them, He will put none of the diseases upon them He brought upon the Egyptians (disobedient world).[2] Not one of His commandments tells us not to eat clean meat. Neither did God say that if we do, we will become ill as Christian vegetarian leaders are preaching these days.

---

[1] 1 Tim. 4:1-6

[2] Today millions of God's people are sick, but perhaps not from diseases He put upon them. If the poor health is due to poor diet, both the world and Christians will suffer the same.

On the contrary, Genesis 9:3, Leviticus 11, Deuteronomy 12:15, 1 Corinthians 10:25, 1 Timothy 4:3, Proverbs 27:27, and other Scriptures have commanded God's people *to* eat these foods since the flood at least. In the 1 Timothy 4 passage above, the Holy Spirit specifically warns against vegetarianism/veganism in the last days in which we live.

The Apostle Paul referred to those who did not eat meat as being weak in the faith, and having a weak conscience, even when some refused to eat meat offered to idols.[1] Yet they still had other animal-based foods such as wild game, fish, chicken, butter, milk, and eggs.

Doctrines Of Devils:

Gordon Tessler, PhD, Christian nutrition scientist, presents the truth clearly, as follows: "Whether eating that which God commands us *not* to eat…or not eating that which God commanded us *to* eat, both are "doctrines of devils."[2] In 1 Timothy 4 above, the Scripture specifically associates commanding to abstain from meat with doctrines of demons.

Eating is more than assuaging hunger, enjoying what tastes good, and social interaction. Based upon disobedience, deception, and rebellion against God's plan for eating after the Fall, veganism, whether with non-Christians or Christians, is an exceedingly serious matter to the Creator, and increasingly to this nation.

Since Satan deceived Eve with the fruit,[3] food has been a powerful tool for his destruction of God's creatures. His testing of hungry Jesus in the wilderness with bread, was another clever attempt to inflict pain on the Almighty. That fallen angel thought he had destroyed mankind forever when Eve obeyed him, unaware that God would provide His very Son to save man. Had Jesus done as Satan suggested and turned the stone into bread,[4] He would have come under the enemy's dominion, and we would be

---

[1] Rom. 14:1-2, 1 Cor. 8:4, 7; 1 Cor. 10
[2] Gen. 3:17, 1 Tim. 4:1-5
[3] 1 Tim. 2:14
[4] Luke 4:3

eternally lost as the devil desired.

Food has powerful potential and long-term spiritual effects. We see our enemy's hand in mankind's eating and food from Eden to this end time, e.g., Genesis 3, Daniel 1, 1 Corinthians 10, 1 Timothy 4:1-4, *et al.*[1] Therefore, God gave us commandments to guide us so that we too are not deceived in the last days.

"Touch not, taste not," vegetarian/vegan leaders demand. "Come and dine!" was Jesus' invitation to His disciples! At the Last Supper, He confided His passion to eat that Passover lamb with His disciples. God ate veal while seated before Abraham and Sarah.

It is in Satan's interest to affect the health of God's children in particular, including extreme diets – from the PD to veganism. There are eventual health losses to individuals who follow them, and overall loss to the kingdom of God's dear Son; regardless of whether the movements/cults are led by apostates or simply by the deceived. God is opposed to false doctrine, including false dietary doctrine which diminishes and rejects His commandments and gifts.

Responsibilities Of The Leaders & The Led

Veganism encompasses a wide variety of people groups, including but not limited to certain Christians, New Age,[2] Eastern and other religions, groups with no particular religion, such as teen agers, and other groups, all of whom have their "expert" leaders.

Quite a number of pastors today don't seem to have been taught the whole Word. They are being grossly misled by strong, likewise deceived leaders promoting so-called "Biblical nutrition" that definitely is not. Probably most of those spreading and receiving false doctrine, do not themselves know what the Bible teaches about God's plan for eating after the Fall, and have little or no education in whole foods nutrition science. Some, including followers, may perish for lack of knowledge. "If the blind follow the blind, they will both fall into the ditch," the axiom warns.

With years of appearances before large audiences of the easy

---

[1] Fasting denies a door of temptation during prayer.
[2] Some of the largest churches today are New Age teaching.

to lead "sheep," including mega-churches, TV, and radio, plus their books with impressive endorsements by unknowing nationally known figures, these Christian "nutrition expert" identities may become enmeshed with the "doctrine of demons" they proclaim.

If such influentials are not humble, don't take time to get alone with Almighty God - whose nutrition plan they have grossly distorted, maligned, and trampled – until He reveals His truth and themselves to them, they will not...they *cannot,* repent. They must answer to God for that which they do with their influence.

Yet, deceived followers have a responsibility as well. "All we like sheep have gone astray; we have turned every one to his own way, and the Lord has laid on Him the *iniquity* of us all," Isaiah 53:6 puts it. The rebellious song writer declared, "I did it my way..." Please note Scripture calls this "iniquity." It *always* gets us in trouble.

The "Bottom Line"

God's principles are an extension of himself, who He is. Satan is not a creator, but a perverter, e.g., Scripture, sex, music, and foods, including principles in God's Word regarding these and others. The Prudent Diet and vegetarianism /veganism, have in common the rejection of God's full plan for eating after the Fall. To varying degrees, these diets renounce foods blessed and commanded by God. Being thankful for and enjoying His gifts according to 1 Timothy 4:4, protects us from rebellion, and the Deceiver's inadequate alternatives.

God's Plan B

When those who have suffered ill effects from vegetarian/vegan diets, then have their eyes opened to significant truth, they often have a zeal to help others see the liberating light. That is good. However, with little or no formal education in the science of nutrition, they sometimes go on to put together new diets they claim to be "God's complete diet," "the only diet that always works," "the perfect diet," and other like claims.

Some may be surprised to learn there has been no perfect diet since Eden, including God's plan for eating after the Fall. Even if there were, the perfect foods are not available for it. Imperfect bodies all react and respond differently in varying degrees to various foods for various reasons. We must therefore speak in generalities and principles to some degree in respect to eating after the Fall.

Even foods mentioned in the Bible (including many other foods discussed in the coming companion book to this one), may not be tolerated by each body due to sensitivities and food allergies. Please understand that only pre-Fall earth was perfect. What we have had ever since is *Plan B*, not the Creator's best that was rejected and traded for a single, whatever kind of fruit. However, *this divine provision is the best we now have for most people.*

Thousands of years after Eden, sinful man has polluted the earth, depleted the soil, devitalized his food, and made himself chronically ill. With our increasing toxic load (endogenous and exogenous) and genome aberations, and with earth itself winding down, every individual is only relatively well at best.

Dietarily doing our best, means eating animal-based and other nutrient-dense, foods, phytonutrient rich plant foods, broths, cultured foods (yogurt and raw saukraut are examples), and whole foods concentrates (rather than synthetic, fractionated isolates for the most part).[1] *Then* in faith, we can ask God to "take up the slack," so to speak, to "pat it all in place."

I cannot tell you that if you follow God's plan for eating for most of us today, that you will not get sick ever again. I *can* say that based upon my personal and professional experience, you likely will not become ill nearly as often. My husband stopped having colds and flu when he stopped eating at the world's table at work and on the way. We did not suffer a contagious disease in decades until I prepared this manuscript for a bound book. Go figure…

Profound stress of a major move, extensive renovation of the new property, dealing for over 18 months with disingenuous contractors, landscaping of a quarter acre, high level of ozone for

---

[1] Nutriceuticals may sometimes be advisable in pharmacological dosages.

over a year due to faulty installation of an electronic air filter, and of course, nutritional consultations besides the usual research, newspaper column, and book writing – surely took their toll at our ages, in spite of all that could be done nutritionally. (Who knows where we would be without it?) Yet a very comprehensive test showed my mineral and extensive trace mineral levels to be exceptionally normal.

Besides an excellent fresh, whole foods diet and whole foods concentrates, we also practice common-sense prevention. While we are not paranoid, we avoid unnecessary winter crowds where people are coughing, sneezing, and shaking hands. When we go out, we wash our hands upon returning home (store door handles, carts, money, and other things that countless people touch, carry all sorts of pathogens).

Some people have food allergies and insensitivities to various foods. Some will be able to eat only small or no amounts of certain of God's good foods (that's not His fault). This long after Eden, we all have individual weaknesses and health challenges we were born with or developed afterward, that affect how the body processes foods and nutrients. Yet for many, the level of wellness is improved, a high level safely maintained for the long-term.

Though there are many variables in even this diet, depending upon the individual and availability of certain foods, we *all* require the same nutrients, some more, some less. Without question, God's plan for eating after Eden has the most nutrients of any diet.

Listen to your body; educate yourself, especially with the resources that whole foods nutrition science offers when it agrees with scriptural principles, and your body.[1] As needed and when they are available, working with qualified whole-foods practitioners who are informed in these principles and experienced, can be of great benefit. Especially must we seek guidance from Him who designed us, the whole foods, and the plan.

A Far Better Solution

At the time we purchased the three year old Angus we called "Big Mama," she had already produced two calves, had one at her

---

[1] Including the use of Resources at the end of this book.

side, and had been bred back. In other words, she was nursing while carrying another calf. She was eating for three.

That winter I noticed she was wheezing. Our cattle manager thought it was not a problem, but it wasn't good either. When we sold our vastly improved land after 28 years, organic grass-fed Big Mama had raised the calf she came with, had easily given birth to the one she was carrying when we bought her, and raised it well. She had done an outstanding job of producing with no need for meds as long as we had her. I so appreciated her and her performance in response to our care, I refused to breed her back; insisting that the new owner allow her to rest a year. He did. Commercial dairymen say they cannot afford to do that. However, their cattle have shorter life spans, and require pharmaceuticals.

If the reason for avoiding animal foods is because of the farming and meat industries' malpractices in care, slaughter, and land use, why not promote and practice compassionate, organic animal husbandry, while greatly improving the land as we did for decades? Why "throw the baby out with the bathwater" just to get rid of the "dirty water"? Scripture teaches compassionate, humane treatment with proper nutrition for animals; good conservation, as well as periodic resting of animals, farm land, and fruit trees. Like sex and music, food - including animal-based food - becomes unhealthy when God's principles and commandments are perverted or averted, whether in growing food or eating it. At the same time, difficult times, we must seek out sources of the Creator's wholesome foods – in the countryside, or on the Internet if need be.

Linda's Restoration

Vegetarians account for fewer than 10% of Americans; yet 80% of vegetarians are also said to suffer from ulcerative colitis, Crohn's disease, and other inflammatory bowel diseases. It is not difficult to understand why bowel diseases are associated with osteoporosis, and impaired nutrient absorption, including fat-soluble vitamins from animal-based foods required for healthy bones and much else. Our bodies are unaware of the many and various philosophies and religions; they simply crave these God-given resources.

My friend, Linda, a vegetarian and health food store nutrition consultant, suffered chronic diarrhea and other symptoms from inflammatory bowel disease (IBD). Unable to tolerate the high insoluble fiber diet of veganism, and with consistent encouragement, she finally decided to add meat to her diet for tissue healing and rebuilding.

Shortly thereafter she shared with me, "It tasted soooooooo good! My body was absolutely *thrilled* with the first bite, as though it was finally getting what it so desperately needed! I am doing much better already."

It took only a little meat to make a "believer" out of her! Today she is a certified nutritionist teaching fresh, whole-foods nutrition that includes flesh foods. She is but one walking proof that it works!

There are many more "reformed" vegetarians than you might think, including one popular radio talk show host and medical doctor. This book includes more of those restoration stories in testimony to the wisdom of our Creator.

Shall We Go Backward Or Look Forward?

We can never go back to the garden where life began on this earth. Yet, without question we *can* do a great deal to improve and maintain our wellness level and quality of life; to avoid premature death so that we may "occupy" (work for God) until the day of His Son and our Savior's appearing.

In the interim, we are not looking back to Eden, but forward to eternity with our risen Lord. We look forward to that day when there will be again be no sickness, pain, sorrow or death, when we will enjoy glorified bodies, and eat from the tree the first Adam did not value.

> "Blessed are those who do His commandments, that they may have the right to the Tree of Life, and may enter through the gates into the City."[1]

---

[1] Rev. 22:15

Romans 14: Peace Making Priority

The Apostle Paul said that not all have the same understanding of what is a healthy diet. The vegan is weak in the faith, he said; however, we are not to offfend or break fellowship over eating matters. "Let not him who eats [meat] despise him that eats [it] not; and let not him which eats not [meat] judge him that eats [meat] for God has received him."

When I am with brethren who do not have knowledge of nutrition science and the Scriptures for understanding regarding this, if they ask and are open to truth, I sometimes teach them, or tell them about this book. However, I find it almost impossible to convince vegan Christians of certain leaders until they are motivated by conditions resulting from their dietary deficiencies, e.g. muscle loss. Though veganism won't send us to hell, the physiological consequences remain. If they are not ready, I do not mention nutrition, though I do not eat the non-foods they may enjoy. We fellowship as fellow believers in the Lord Jesus Christ.

Paul taught that eating meat is not wrong. To the contrary, we are commanded to eat certain meat and dairy products. Yet if someone believes meat-eating is a sin, to *him* it *is* sin, though not to others who eat it. "...He that doubts is damned if he eats [meat] because he eats not of faith, for whatsoever is not of faith is sin...Let us therefore follow after the things which make for peace,[1] and things wherewith one may edify another."

Meat: It's Here To Stay

Meat eating will be part of God's people's diet into the Millennium. Isaiah 25:6 and 66:10-24 reveal that at that time God will make a feast for *all* His people (not just the Jews), that will include choice pieces of meats with very nutritious bone marrow.[2]

How will today's Christians who refuse to eat meat, respond on that great feast day? Will they abstain with a quiet "No, thank you"? Perhaps finally, they will no longer be afraid of meat when their Creator Himself serves it to them! Who in that great and

---

[1] See also 1 Co. 7:15.
[2] Dan. 7:14, Isa. 66:10-23

glorious crowd would dare to question what is served, or tell the Master "No thank you," or that which He is serving is a "killer food"? More importantly, will God accommodate their choices not found on His menu? From Scripture quoted here besides other passages, it does not appear so.

The following letter by Susan Siemers of Indiana, appears at the USDA website. Her heart surgeon disclosed the fact of the perfect condition of her arteries after Siemers consumed meat and dairy fats for decades. To those aware of the growing body of scientific evidence substantiating same, this comes as no surprise. [1]

USDA
Nutrition and Your Health:
Dietary Guidelines for Americans
2005 Dietary Guideline Committee Report

To the Dietary Guidelines Advisory Committee:

Summary

The data do not support a positive correlation between cardiac disease and saturated fat consumption. My health history is a case in point, as I was raised eating very few sweets, but much milk, cream and butter, and my arteries are free of plaque, in spite of a "high" cholesterol count.

Comments

...I was born on a farm, married a farmer, drank whole milk (unpasteurized), [ate] butter, and...a lot of meat. My cholesterol has always been around 225, give or take 10 points. In today's world, that is considered high and my last three doctors have all tried to get me to take statins. My triglycerides are very low (below 75).

Well, I am lucky (or unlucky, depending on how you look at it), in that I have a genetic disease, fibromuscular dysplasia. The muscles in the wall of the artery wrap around the artery like a rubber band, causing a stenosis. In my case, I have three stenoses, with small aneurysms behind them. It is in my right renal artery,

---

[1] health.gov/dietaryguidelines/dga2005/comments/ViewAll.asp#4

and it was discovered several months after my normally low (100/60) blood pressure jumped to 230/130 in a one week period and resisted all treatment with hypertension medication. Angioplasty seems to have taken care of it.

Here is why I am lucky. During the second angioplasty (they cautiously did one stenosis at a time in 1988), the doctor who was performing the angioplasty took a look at my arteries all the way to my heart. He was amazed at them, saying they were totally free of plaque. So my high fat diet - AND a cholesterol reading that is considered too high - has caused absolutely no injuries to my arteries.

The reason I say I am lucky is that I have an iron-clad argument about why I should not be on statins. (By the way, 50% of people who have heart attacks have normal cholesterol levels. That does not mean we need to lower cholesterol even further - what it may indicate is that cholesterol level is a poor indicator of heart health.)

Having this disease has caused me to do a great deal of research. I am amazed at how we have latched on to a low fat diet when all the data say that we need to limit sugar and simple carbohydrates, not fat. Granted, we must be fussy about our fats, but **the very fats I was loading up on as a child were the right ones**. What happened? Why were they denigrated?

I am totally NOT convinced by any recent trials that are conducted and paid for by the very pharmaceutical companies that will benefit from the sale of statin drugs. If we look at the "old" data, they just simply do not support a low fat diet. In fact, to the contrary, they indicate a high fat diet is better for us.

I was a vegetarian for 15 years. On average, I probably ate about 700 g of carbohydrates a day, and did try to watch my fats. During that time, my teeth fell apart (two bridges, lots of crowns, root canals), I developed hypoglycemia and diverticulosis, and I begin struggling with my weight. I also developed some pretty nasty mood swings.

Then I read a book, *Life Without Bread, How A Low Carb Diet Can Save Your Life*,[1] and decided to go back to eating meat

---

[1] Allan & Lutz. See Resources

and fat. Since giving up my vegetarian ways in late 2000, my hypoglycemia is virtually symptomless, my bowels are working right again and I have had no additional problems with my teeth. My weight has stabilized. My mood swings are still with me, but I guess four out of five ain't bad!

Please go back to the data provided in the 1950 **Seven Country Study.** Nothing in that study supported a low fat diet. There was no correlation strong enough between fat consumption and heart health to raise a concern.

What SHOULD have raised concern was the fact that in some of the countries, increased fat intake actually LOWERED the incidence of death rates due to heart disease. That should have spurred the researchers to find out why it varied so greatly from country to country. The clue is in one paragraph in the middle of this 200-page report. It states that **sugar intake is correlated with heart disease**. No difference country to country, over all this correlation held true. So why didn't the researches look at those countries with high fat intake AND high incidence of heart disease and look at their sugar consumption? I don't know. I am hoping that your committee will take a look at this now. Certainly the proof is in the pudding.

Since 1950, when we were told fats were bad and margarine was good, since we began replacing the good-tasting fat in food with sugar to mask its bland taste, diabetes has risen to epidemic proportions, as has obesity. The answer is not to do what we have been doing since 1950 only more so (even less fat), but to look back at how we were eating prior to 1950.

I implore you to examine historical data regarding the correlation between overall health and fat consumption, and to look with great suspicion at recent data compiled by drug companies that have a vested interest in the outcome of these studies. The health of our nation is at stake, and it should be examined without the taint of politics and corporate interests.

Respectfully,
Susan Siemers Walkerton, IN 46574
Submission Date: September 23, 2004

health.gov/dietaryguidelines/dga2005/comments/ViewAll.asp#4

10

Meat, Fish & Fowl - Should We Eat Them All?

An Unforgettable Object Lesson

On the Gulf Coast where I grew up, seafood is abundant. One summer my aunt and uncle loaned my family the use of their bay cottage. When the tide was out at night, one of the older children held the lantern while Daddy gigged for flounder. During the day we staked a chicken carcass further down the sandy shore; and after a time in the hot sun, it was rank! The blue crabs gathered to feast on the decomposing chicken. We easily caught these shellfish for a big crab boil, greatly enjoying fried crab claws by the platter.

While working my way through undergrad school, I was accounting secretary to the treasurer for a large corporation which employed barges for transporting of cargo. One day a group of us were enjoying our lunches, when a barge captain came in, sat down, and told us of the latest accident. He said one of the laborers had fallen from his barge about two weeks previous and disappeared in the strong undertow before he could be rescued.

The captain went on to say that the decomposing body had been discovered on the river bank that warm morning - covered with big blue crabs. I didn't eat crabs for a long time...

Unclean Means Unfit For Human's To Eat

After years of Bible study, I have come to believe certain animals were, and still are unclean; not because of the law, but the other way around. In other words, God's law declared them unclean because they actually *are* unclean and unhealthy for us humans to eat.

In Leviticus 11 and Deuteronomy 14, God gives us His meat "shopping lists." You may say, and I would agree with you, that most of today's Church believes those lists were ceremonial law which was fulfilled with the crucifixion. Therefore, they are not for us today, these Christians reason. Though only clean meat was offered for sacrifices, these chapters have directly to do with what we are to eat and not eat. Whether they were or were not part of that law, is not relevant to our discussion here.

Another example of avoiding uncleanness is given in Deuteronomy 23:13-14. In this passage, God's people are commanded to relieve themselves outside the camp in a specified area, employing a particular implement to dig a hole for their excrement, which was referred to as "unclean" – not ceremonially, but actually.[1] In the text, unclean means *unclean*.

Contrast this with Third World countries today, where latrines are virtually non-existent outside the cities, and defecation occurs near living quarters and along drainage ditches, contaminating bathing and drinking water as well. More than 80% of diseases in Ethiopia and some other countries is linked to poor sanitation.

God's people had the first sewage disposal plan, about six thousand years ahead of today's. Jesus did not fulfill the Deuteronomy 23:14 law when He was sacrificed. God's sanitation principles continue today because powerful pathogens haven't ceased.

By the same principle, avoiding unclean animals is not a matter of legalism and ceremonial law for us; but a matter of health and welfare, life and death.

Jesus' blood makes men clean when they believe in His sacrificial death, but the crucifixion did nothing for unclean

---

[1] "...[T]herefore your camp shall be holy [clean], that He see no unclean thing among you," the text commands. "For God has not called us to uncleanness, but unto holiness," Paul told the New Testament Church.[1] In Leviticus 13, holiness is also associated with eating clean foods. ("Cleanliness is next to godliness," we were taught as children getting our ears washed.)

animals. You might then ask, "If we are not to eat such, then why *did* God create them?"

The Creator's Purpose For Unclean Animals

Many years after the barge captain told his story about the blue crabs on the putrefying corpse, God began teaching me His plan for nutrition after the Fall, and brought to mind that example. With the thought came the explanation: it was precisely to maintain cleanliness that *un*clean animals were created!

The Creator's purpose for most unclean animals is to be His scavengers, His "garbage collectors" or "sanitation workers" of land and sea.[1] Their role has not changed since Eden. In fact, as His "housekeepers," they are more necessary than ever in our ecology. Created as such, they have been unclean from the beginning; not just since Moses' law.

In Matthew 24:28 we are told eagles clean up carcasses. We sometimes see buzzards zooming down and quickly disposing of "road kill;" shell fish working to clean up beaches and coastal waters by filtering pollution and contaminants, and eating dead things.

Many scavenger sea animals have been assigned the task of keeping the oceans clean. Hogs - classic omnivores – help control disease-carrying vermin numbers; clean up dead animals and animal manure; and all manner of putrefaction and rottenness. Earthworms help process decaying plant matter below ground.

Again, the question is this: did the earth cease to need all these sanitation workers with Jesus' death? Or could it be that with five billion people on this planet, we need them more than ever?

Further, can we now healthfully eat animals that feed on corruption of the worst sort? Most Americans – Christians and non-Christians - ignore the difference between what God created

---

[1] Not all unclean animals are scavengers, e.g. rabbits and horses are not. However, horse meat may be infected with viruses and parasites. Rabbits (Guinea pigs and rats) recycle feces, eating some directly from their anuses for extra vitamin B_{12}. Rabbits are carriers of tularemia (rabbit fever), a bacterial disease.

for our nourishment and what He made for "taking out the garbage."

Ever so often news reports warn against eating contaminated shellfish (feeding on shoreline pollution). When we were in Puerto Rico, the ocean water at the Ponce beach was polluted such that swimming was not allowed. However, I noticed tourists ate the toxic shellfish from that water.

We should not eat plants feeding on toxic substances. Nor should we consume animals that feed on pathogenic diets. "We are what we eat," is often heard, and *so are animals*.

Pigs In Contrast

When the Prodigal Son repented, he left pigs and returned to a fatted calf. Abraham served veal to holy angels and God. Peter spoke of the unclean dog returning to its vomit and the hog wallowing in filthy mud. Throughout the Word, in the Old and New Testaments we find contrasts of clean and unclean. Here's one more:

After multiplying the loaves and fish to feed the multitudes, the compassionate Jesus had the disciples take up the leftovers on more than one occasion; doubtless He gave them to the people to take home with them. In contrast, we have the story of the Gadarene who lived in tombs with literal unclean, decomposing bodies as a result of his being possessed by unclean spirits. When Jesus cast out the demons, they preferred to move into hogs, not because those animals were ceremonially unclean, but actually. In granting the demons' request, the same compassionate Jesus got rid of tons of pork rather than give the unclean meat to people.[1] Surely He had in mind some of the following health issues put forth by professor and medical doctor, Hans-Heinrich Reckeweg:[2]

...[S]uffering from biliary gallstones, inflammations of the appendix, inevitable gain in weight, high blood

---

[1] Mark 5.11-13 and Luke 8.32-33
[2] Reckeweg H-H, The Adverse Influence of Pork Consumption On Health, *Biological Therapy,* Vol 1 No 2:1983

pressure, fatty degeneration of the liver, or other dreaded diseases, particularly arthritis and arthrosis, [as] a direct result of pork consumption...

...[I]nflammations of the appendix and gall bladder, biliary colics, acute intestinal catarrh, gastroenteritis with typhoid and paratyphoid symptoms, as well as acute eczema, carbuncles, sudoriparous abscesses, and other [skin issues related to toxins]. These symptoms can [also] be observed after consuming sausage meats (including salami which contains pieces of bacon in the form of fat.

All these and more diseases are associated with the sutoxins (toxic and stress factors) in pork according to Professor Reckeweb.[1] We will look at others further on in this chapter.

Interestingly, I noted porcine-related diseases includes carbuncles (very large, painful boils with heavy cores) from toxins. I recall that when my mother was pregnant with my younger sister Mother craved pickled pigs' feet, and ate them by the jar at one sitting. She suffered from terrible carbuncles which never recurred after she ceased eating pork. But that may be the least of the adverse effects of this meat according to Dr. Reckeweb and other experts.

Horrifying Risks Of The 21st Century

Ancient medical papyri, with recipes and spells for a large variety of diseases and ailments, include one for trichinae, the pig parasite.[2] It has not gone away. The federal government's Center For Disease Control (CDC) warns at its website (cdc.gov): "Do not allow hogs to eat uncooked carcasses of other animals, including rats, which may be infected with trichinellosis." Referring to the coming Millennium, we have interesting unfulfilled prophecies in Isaiah 65 and 66 regarding pigs and vermin.[3]

---

[1] http://reactor-core.org/pork-consumption.html
[2] Baily N, 2002, Ancient Egyptian Medicine; mnsu.edu/emuseum/prehistory/egypt/dailylife/medicine2.htm; Ead HA, *Medicine in Old Egypt;* levity.com/alchemy/islam22.html
[3] Isa. 66:17. In vs. 23, note the text refers to "all," not only Jews.

Yet little is said about that devastating parasite from pork. In fact, most Americans believe we now raise hogs on clean concrete that is washed down and we don't have to worry about *Trichinella spiralis* anymore. Hogs still eat vermin with parasites (dangerous to humans) that enter the pigs' restrictive enclosures, or they may be exposed other ways. Yet trichinosis is not the worst concern if the following information is only a fraction factual. According to Alix Fano, Director of the Campaign For Responsible Transplantation (CRT),

> Porcine tissues and cells used for transplants are not "purified" and may contain a host of porcine viruses that are **part of the pig genome and cannot not be bred out.** These include viruses that are known as well as those that have yet to be identified...[1]
>
> There is no way to screen for viruses that are not yet known. Proceeding with xenotransplantation could expose patients and **non-patients** to a host of new animal viruses that could remain dormant for months or years before being detected...
>
> This "risk of infecting patients and **the general public** with viruses from pigs genetically altered to carry human genes - biotechnology companies' source animals of choice for cells, tissues, and organs," is very real according to CRT. In fact, genetically engineered animals are more susceptible to a host of diseases because of weaker immune systems...

This coalition of 90 international public interest groups representing over two million members, believes that cross-species transplants should be banned. At least 16 patients have died during or after receiving such transplants and/or pig cell injections into their brains. There are a number of grave concerns; however, please note the life-threatening risks here are not restricted to patients participating in these highly lucrative experiments the FDA protects.

The following disturbing information from press releases of

---

[1] Fano A, Dir, CRT, personal communication, June 13, 2007

the CRT[1] reminds us of the wisdom of God in long ago designating pigs as unclean, not to be touched by humans, much less the internalizing of their organs and cells in human transplantation. Swine flu, viruses, and other infections are still highly lethal for the general population, warns CRT:

> There are over 25 diseases from pigs that can infect humans and new ones keep surfacing, including Porcine Reproductive and Respiratory Syndrome virus, and paramyxovirus. The "Nipah" virus, discovered in Malaysia...spread from pigs to humans, infecting 229 people - causing high fever, aches, and convulsions, killing 111, and leading to the mass slaughter of 640,500 pigs. The CDC...said the virus had "never been seen before." A similar illness afflicted 11 slaughterhouse workers in Singapore...That may be why researchers at the Mayo Clinic [tested] 300 slaughterhouse workers in the U.S. for signs of infection by pig viruses, including the Porcine Endogenous Retroviruses (PERVs), found throughout the pig genome, that have infected human cells in test tubes.
>
> The influenza virus of 1918, which resembled a common swine flu, killed more people in modern history than any other epidemic including AIDS and the Black Plague. A new influenza strain (H3N2), which swept across Northern China to Hong Kong last year, **has been spreading among U.S. pig herds.**
>
> ...But a year-long (sic) study on a small group of patients is not proof of safety, or efficacy. The Novartis/CDC study, among other things, fails to account for long disease latency periods.
>
> Indeed, a January 20, 1999, study in the Journal of the National Cancer Institute reported that Simian Virus 40, (SV40), which contaminated polio vaccine in the early 1960s, was regarded as harmless, until recently. Scientists now say that initial studies may not have been conducted over a long enough period, and new highly

---

[1] crt-online.org.

sensitive tests have detected the presence of SV40 in different types of human tumors, perhaps responsible for 1,000 new human cancers each year. [This vaccine may also have been linked to chronic fatigue, appearing 30 years later.]

"History could repeat itself if we allow xenotransplants to go forward. The new Public Health Service guidelines on xenotransplantation...will never eliminate risk, and no pig will ever be virus-free," says CEO Fano.

The FDA, which has approved...clinical xenotransplant trials, has admitted that xenotransplantation is dangerous. Leading virologists and FDA officials have acknowledged that the technology could transmit known and unknown animal viruses to patients, their families, health care workers, and **the public at large**, possibly triggering an AIDS-like pandemic...[1]

Viruses that are harmless to their animal hosts, can be deadly when transmitted to humans...Many viruses, as innocuous as the common cold or as lethal as Ebola, can be transmitted via a mere cough or sneeze. An animal virus residing in a xenograft recipient could become airborne, infecting scores of people, and causing a potentially deadly viral epidemic of global proportions...[2]

Sure, we're told to cook pork until well done. Does that necessarily mean all microbes will be destroyed? Do you know what temperature and how long is required to kill each kind of virus, bacteria, or whatever else may have come with the chops or roast? [3] If you cook pork ribs to "well done" at 325 degrees, and your neighbor bar-b-ques his, do you know if the parasites are also "well done" in either? I don't. I *do* know that well done meat is

---

[1] crt-online.org/lawsuit.html
[2] crt-online.org/wrong.html
[3] Large white worms (Ascaris Suum) 250 to 400 mm long are often found in sows' and finishing pigs' feces. These female worms produce 500.000 to 1 mil. eggs per day, that survive outside the pig for many years. They are resistant to drying and freezing. (Pigsite.com)

difficult to digest, and its protein denatured, making for poor utilization by humans.

Dr. Olympio Pinto, Rio de Janeiro, Brazil, noted "profound reaction" in live red blood cells one hour after patients eat pork, during which a disturbing percentage of red blood cells became "...what are termed 'ghosts'...red blood cells that have lost their hemoglobin, resulting in a lack of oxygen transport.[1]

Poisonous Pig Pollution

"Hog slurry (manure and urine mixture) is about 100 times more toxic than raw human sewage," according to Brandon University biologist, Bill Paton.[2] Where is it coming from? A single mega barn stuffs in 125,000 sows for bringing two and a half million pigs to market annually.[3] (With such conditions, we immediately think of antibiotics, leading to resistant strains of bacteria.) Like the transplantation business, pork is very big business.

With Eva Pip's home place surrounded by livestock factory farms, she heaps scorn on the industry's PR machine:

> How ironic that a recent television commercial produced by the pork industry, drives home this point. We see a pretty picture of contented pigs, unrestrained and outdoors in the sunshine, while a cute little girl is helping to distribute the pigs' food with her own adorable hands. Yet this is the very producer that the hog industry is destroying...Why does the industry not show its real face

---

[1] Huggins HA, *It's All In Your* Head, *Diseases Caused By Silver-Mercury Fillings*, Life Sciences Press, 1990-63 Dr. Huggins explains in his book that the body may produce replacement cells within a relatively short time, however, not without impact.

[2] Baumel S, Hog Wild, Manitoba's Wreckless Agriventure, *The Aquarian*, Summer 2004
aquarianonline.com/Values/hogwild.html

[3] Small family farms of every kind are almost gone. Huge factory-farms buy up all competition, or the small producer is squeezed out of the market when he can no longer compete. The small farmer has minimal adverse environmental impact since livestock are well spaced. The comparatively small amount of waste causes small localized problems.

— the sows confined in tight barren crates, standing on their own filth, breathing noxious fumes, with the only sunlight they will ever see being the time when they are crammed into the transports to go to slaughter? Would a little girl be helping to feed thousands of pigs in such a place? It would be child abuse...[1]

Concerning Chicken...

Chicken is included herein with quality protein. Though they are included in the Bible in a few places, they are not listed in Leviticus 11 and Deuteronomy 14. Chickens are not birds of prey (unclean), and they eat grass when given the opportunity. However, they are not herbivorous like clean animals listed there. Actually, they are omnivores, and may be considered to be at least somewhat scavengers. We have seen them eat unclean things of various sorts.

Some – not all - organic chickens, including layers, are fed chiefly corn and soy, with no greens at all. A few organic chicken producers feed a diet without soy, and/or provide green pasture.

I do not have a definitive word on this food. Today's Jewish community considers chicken to be clean. Jesus described eggs as good gifts; He did not add, "but do not eat chickens."

"Cleanliness Is Next To Godliness"

"For God has not called us to uncleanness, but unto holiness," Paul told the New Testament Church.[1] "Cleanliness is next to godliness," we were assured as children getting our ears washed. In Leviticus 13, holiness is also associated with eating clean foods.

Beginning with Genesis, the loving Father has been sanctifying and calling to Himself those who are righteous. "...[K]now that the Lord has set apart him that is godly for Himself," the Psalmist declared.[2] This process involves the whole man, including the physical body.

---

[1] Baumel S, *Loc. cit.*
[2] Psa. 4:3a

And the very God of peace sanctify you **wholly;** and I pray God your **whole spirit and soul and body** be preserved blameless unto the coming of our Lord Jesus Christ.

In the original, "preserved" means to guard from loss or injury. This includes the physical body as part of the whole man God created. He cares about it, and what affects it as His temple. He put unclean foods off base for us, thousands of years before anyone knew the risks of pork and other unclean meat. "Moreover by them [His law, statutes, fear of the Lord] is Thy servant warned: and in keeping of them there is great reward."[1] Do you suppose these "great rewards" may include what we *don't* get!

1 Timothy 4:1-6: End Time Errors

We have looked at this passage from other perspectives. Here Paul, the apostle, confirmed God's plan for eating after the Fall, including Leviticus 11, had not changed in four thousand years. Furthermore, it would be valid two thousand years later in our day. Let's now turn our attention to his very important warning - God's warning - to the end time Church:

1. The Spirit speaks expressly that in the latter times some shall depart from the faith, giving heed to seducing spirits, and doctrines of devils;
2. Speaking lies in hypocrisy; having their consciences seared with a hot iron;
3. Forbidding to marry and commanding to abstain from meats [*bromatone*] **which God has created to be received** with thanksgiving of them which believe and know the truth.
4. For every creature of God is good and nothing to be refused if it be received with thanksgiving.
5. For it is **sanctified** by the **Word of God** and prayer.
6. If thou put the brethren in remembrance of these things, thou shalt be a good minister of Jesus Christ,

---

[1] Psa. 19:11

nourished up in the words of faith and of good doctrine, whereunto thou has attained.

Most Chrisians then and now, would not agree they should eat no meat at all, as the aforementioned apostates demand. Many brethren *do*, however, believe this text teaches the other extreme - eating *any* kind of meat. Here we have another synecdoche where a part is referred to as the whole. It is written to those who knew the truth and ate only clean foods.

Actually, only those animals "which God created to be received" are referenced. They are to be eaten by those who also believe and know the truth regarding foods He *set apart* (sanctified) by His Word. There was only the Old Testament at the time Paul wrote this. Shrimp, pork, squid, and skunk, were not sanctified by that word nor Paul's.[1]

If we are to eat any and all flesh foods, then how are they set apart? Why do we need to follow that doctrine *carefully* if we can eat every kind of meat? And which meats are those?[2] That passage does not end at verse three.

They are meats from the clean animals of verse four that God "created to be received (verse three);" those that eat green, living foods - not scavengers that eat disease-carrying vermin, feces, rotten carcasses (carrion) and garbage laden with maggots, flies, and pathogens. The "Word of God" did not sanctify (set apart) unclean animals that were not created to be eaten.

The Apostle Paul wrote that the Holy Spirit spoke this to him specifically regarding the end time – our time, as a "heads up." *What is the Holy Spirit warning us about today?* Vegetarianism – eating *no* meat; and the *carte blanche* reclassification of unclean foods, eating *all* meat, rather than those God created to be eaten. These are errors of two extremes.[3]

---

[1] Lev. 11 and Deut.14, Psa. 104:14, *et al*

[2] *Bromatone* refers to clean, solid foods in general; however, the word "creature" in the following verse tells us which ones are meant here.

[3] Readers may request a scriptural explanation of Acts 10, Mark 7, Romans 14, and other like passages from eatin_after_eden@wvi.com. We cannot guarantee their availability.

11

End Time Provision – Is It For Real?

Why Do We Need It?

Our food has been grown on depleted oils, sprayed multiple times with pesticides, and often with antifungals before periods of transporting and storage. Afterward all that mistreatment, it is industrially altered for our learned tastes and merchants' rofitability. Soon after harvest it becomes devitalized and denatured; adding a toxic load without corresponding nutritional resources to support the body's work to deal with it.

He Is Faithful

God's Word supplies many examples of His provision in various ways, from Egypt's stored grains during famine, to the fresh oil for the widow at Zeraphat. His eye is even on the sparrow, Jesus said. If needed rain falls on the just and the unjust, should we not expect our Provider to meet the needs of His children? We should, and when we trust and ask Him, He does one way or another. If we are to be about His business,[1] we must be properly nourished.

---

[1] "His business" is different for each of us. If you are called to be an at home mom or executive, that is God's will, the same as being a pastor. I would rather be in the will of God as a janitor, if that were His calling for me; than out of His will as governor.

In Pastor Joey's testimony to God's faithfulness to provide, he explains that rather than sickly saints, healthy ones bring glory to their Father! Organically grown foods are important for that; He is interested in our obtaining what we need for His plan for eating and optimum health.[1]

For nearly 40 years we grew a great deal of our food, organically of course. A couple of times it was only a tomato plant in a pot on a balcony or deck. However, for about 30 years it was a very large garden, eggs, beef and lamb. It was very difficult for me to leave that a couple of years ago when the time came. But He has not forsaken His own even in this provision, and even in old age.

An Amazing End Time Surprise!

After so many years of teaching God's gardening and the eating of fresh whole foods, it seems that almost overnight organic has become very popular! Supermarket chains suddenly moved these fresh foods from a tiny corner to the middle of the newly renovated produce department. It's become "green" to grow this way, and to take care of the earth.

When we moved to the city we of course immediately began to plan a comparatively small garden. I asked the Father for, and we are able to purchase, organic, grass-fed beef, buffalo, and lamb from local farmers who do not feed or treat their animals with antibiotics and other drugs; who raise them humanely and healthfully. Local organic milk and eggs are also abundantly supplied. In only a couple of years it's become so popular we need have no concern about providing the labor and investment to grow it all!

Who would have dreamed this would ever come to pass? Ephesians 3:20 is true, He is indeed able to do exceedingly abundantly above all that we ask or think, according to His power that works within us. City life is far more expensive for us; however, as we have also obeyed His commands regarding

---

[1] There are many good materials exlaining organic gardening and why organic is superior to non-organic.

finances, Father has always provided what we need to purchase these good gifts from His hand.

Whatever The Reason For The Need

There are various reasons people may not have wholesome foods. Sometimes missionaries in other countries must pray over certain foods and trust God to neutralize what isn't healthy. We can do that for cold-water fish. Some must trust God with less than optimum resources while seeking one for organic foods. That is different from simply being unwilling to pay more for real food while spending available funds for unessentials such as movies, cable TV, etc. What are God's priorities for His temple?

Organic grass-fed, flesh foods, butter, milk, cheese, and eggs, are well worth the extra cost when available. It's often a matter of priorities. Good health comes before most things for us.

Tragically, in most states in America today, the government does not allow raw milk in natural foods stores. Most commercial production of animal-based foods cannot be compared with that of local farm products in my opinion. When our local supplier of these good things suddenly switched to beef cattle, I prayed earnestly for nearby pastured eggs and grass-fed raw milk (especially to be used to make raw yogurt). Right away there opened up not one but two local farmers for each! Always, the Creator of these good foods has heard and answered prayer. He is no respecter of persons, His Word promises.

Psalm 78 tells the story of Israel's craving meat, then doubting He could provide it after He had miraculously provided every other need, over and over and over. Even the shoes on their feet never wore out, yet they did not trust in Him. Jesus said, "Ask [believing], that your joy may be made full!"

What About Eating Out?

It is usually impossible to eat organic if one eats out. Not often but sometimes, we may eat attend church dinners, banquets, as guests at others' homes, or a restaurant which offers fresh, whole foods cooked as we wish. We don't say you should never eat out. Select whole foods whenever possible. Then pray over whatever you eat, asking God to remove the toxins, and bless it to the good of your body and His service. Pray also about how often and where you eat out. Whatever you do, do all to the glory of God, Scripture instructs us.

Organically Grown

"Organically grown" on the food label means we are given a two sided advantage: not only are toxic chemicals not used in growing the food, but the fertilizer is divinely created to provide a much higher level of nutrients.

In 2004 Rutgers University released the results of a study showing organic foods have a whopping 300-700 percent more nutrients than non-organically grown foods. In fact, a global plethora of scientific evidence reports that organic foods contain significantly more nutrients than non-organic foods according to the UK's 2007 *999Today* and *Organic Prairie*.[1] The 2003 *Journal of Agriculture and Food Chemistry* reported organically grown berries and corn have 58% more polyphenols, an antioxidant that helps prevent cardiovascular disease; with up to 52% higher levels of vitamin C than the conventionally grown. Soil fertility with balanced nutrients and slower growth makes the difference.[2]

Are organically grown foods worth the extra cost? For us it is in order to avoid the extra load of toxic chemicals. From time immemorial, man consumed his foods organically grown until greed stepped in and perverted them. Of course, as I always emphasize, we should grow our own gardens whenever possible, or at least a few plants or even one tomato or zuchini in the flower bed.

Many books, articles and websites have been devoted to informing us about the serious effects of toxic pesticides and food additives, especially detrimental to our children as well as us. Spend just a little while with one of these informative resources and be convinced forever.

As to organically grown foods' increased levels of nutrients and phytonutrients, to put it in a nutshell, in this endtime our

---

[1] *Organics In The News*, Organic Prairie; *999Today*, Dec. 10, 2007
[2] *Eating Well* magazine, April 2008

bodies need all the support they can get for growth, healing, and prevention of from all we do not wish to suffer. Live life to the maximum, be vigorous and energetic! Eat that which the Creator took the time to provide your body in its purest forms.

Choose Life!

> I call heaven and earth to record this day…that I have set before you life and death…: therefore choose life, that both you and your seed may live.[1]

---

[1] Deut. 30:19

Appendix A [1]

Calcium Absorption:
What Helps, What Hinders

Bone requires more than calcium for formation and maintenance. It contains an abundance of minerals, protein and amino acids, and countless enzymes. Yet calcium is an essential for this.[1]

It works synergistically, and requires many other nutrients for absorption and utilization. As far as we now know, they are as follows: Vitamins A (retinol), B6, B12, folate, C complex, D_3, and K, trace minerals, zinc, copper, silicon, boron, manganese, phosphorous, magnesium, strontium,[2] sulfur, and perhaps others.

Don't expect a pill to include all these, and especially in recommended organic form. A fresh, whole foods diet, plus whole foods concentrates and possibly other supplements are needed to supply them all. Organic whole foods grown in nurtured soils can contribute significantly to providing these multiple nutrients.

Not just nutrients but ratios of calcium in proportion to other minerals are very important. Nutritionists do not agree on the

---

[1] The cheapest form of calcium is carbonate from shell fish or limestone. This form works well for plant nourishment. Some young people may be able to utilize calcium carbonate if stomach acid levels are normal and acid neutralizers aren't ingested. Older people may not absorb this form of calcium efficiently; taking extra amts. of it is like talking louder to someone who doesn't speak your language. Worse, calcium that is not absorbed may be deposited in the body in various unhealthy ways.

[2] Non-toxic strontium, a very important trace mineral (t/m), is not to be confused with strontium 90, the radioactive isotope. Strontium seems to be one of the most effective nutrients for preventing and treating osteoporosis. Chemically similar to calcium, it has been found to replace calcium lacking in bones and teeth, thereby increasing bone density. One study reported by the *New Eng Jnl of Med* of 1,649 post-menopausal women taking this t/m with calcium and vit. D, reported back fracture risk reduced 49% in one year, increasing back bone density by 14%!

calcium/magnesium ratio, as important as it is; however, it is widely accepted that the human body requires 2.5 times more calcium than phosphorous. We see this ideal ratio in sardines with their edible bones. Mother's milk contains a 2.3 calcium/phosphorous ratio.

Certain ingested substances in our time can prevent the building and maintaining of healthy bones. Most soft drinks, and especially colas, are very high in phosphorous.[1] Excessive amounts of this mineral increase urinary calcium excretion. Sugar in such drinks also interferes with calcium and other mineral ratios.

Toxic metal accumulation inhibits bone building as well. Chronic stress diminishes digestion and absorption of nutrients, and especially calcium. In addition to protein digestion, adequate stomach acid is vital for processing calcium.

---

[1] Soft drink consumption by Americans averages more than a gallon weekly.

Appendix B

Pottenger's Cats

Pioneer nutrition scientist Francis Pottenger, MD, conducted a ten year study of forty generations of cats fed various diets as follows: raw meat, and raw milk from cows fed 1) organic grass, 2) organic grass cut and eaten after a day or two, and 3) grain. Other cats were fed 4) cooked, dead diets. Diseases and infertility, killed off the cats on diets 3) and 4), with *shorter and shorter life spans* until the study was ended to prevent losing them all. It took four generations to restore health to the few survivors of the inferior diets, feeding the raw milk and raw meat diet again.

Some claim Dr. Pottenger's study was technically flawed. If so, in principle, it remains valid regardless. God gave us organic, whole, nutrient-dense foods. Man has corrupted these in many ways, leading to ill health and shortened lives. Should He be blamed?

Appendix C

Bob & John's Garden – Far More Than It Appears

Growing a garden is one of the healthiest things you can do for yourself and your family. Whether lecturing or teaching individual patients, I passionately encourage this with one and alls no matter what size you choose. Even one tomato plant contributes an amazing array of nutrients and phytonutrients, some of which no doubt remain yet undiscovered. Together with fresh air, sunshine, and exercise, this activity is very beneficial; especially the way Bob VanDeuzen does it. There's much more to his gardening.

Bob and son John, six year old reflecting his dad's enthusiasm, together grow, cook and eat what they grow. Not only the excellent, organic food, peace and quiet, but also the marvelous camaraderie that has developed during their time together is worth more than words can tell. John will cherish these times alone with Dad in their garden long after Bob is gone, teaching his son Dad's values. Here is Bob's story in his own words.

α α α

"Last night we had the first snow peas of the season, lightly stir-fried in EVOO [extra virgin olive oil], and bit of salt and that's it! Also had a nice salad, and I roasted a chicken. I had gone to the garden with John before and while he picked peas, I clipped rosemary, fresh oregano, and thyme. I made a paste from this with a mortar and pestle along with garlic, salt and pepper and rubbed this mixture under the chicken skin before baking. It was a great meal!

"How pleasing it is for me to gather items from our garden and bring them in to cook. John is a great helper, and he sometimes gets off track while looking at/for bugs or worms while we are working. I could not care less. He also loves the quail family that scoots around by the garden, as well. They are so funny!

"Our property is all-organic of course, and although we have a few more weeds than our neighbors' manicured lawns, I notice our land is full of life. We have lots of birds, bugs, harmless garden snakes, critters, and so forth, while our neighbors' land seems devoid of such things. John spends lots of time outside and I have no problem with him rolling in our grass and playing in our dirt. I would be less inclined to allow him to do so next door!

"Thanks again for all you do and for what you have given me."

Recipes

Delicious, Nutritious, Egg- & Sugar-Free Ice Cream

This is an adaptation such as you can easily do with many recipes, substituting whole foods for counterfeits when possible. We like it best made with fresh goat milk that is naturally homogenized. However, whole cow milk works well also. For those allergic to eggs, it has none. Nor do we use any sugar. The extremely sweet, God-given herb and "dietary supplement," stevia, is all that's needed.[1] A $16 electric ice cream freezer/maker from K-Mart works just fine to give us this economical, nutritious dessert or snack.

Ingredients:

1 qt. goat or whole cow milk
1 c. heavy cream (look for pasteurized rather than ultrapasteurized)
4 T. fresh lemon or limejuice
½ t. sea salt
4 T. Frontier pure vanilla (from HFS, may be omitted if other flavoring used)
½ t. stevia powder

Add all ingredients to ice cream maker/freezer and cover with lid. Place 2" of ice around the canister, then sprinkle ¼ c. of rock salt over it. Continue alternating ice with salt until it reaches the lid. Churn for 15-30 minutes. You may double or triple the recipe to put in the freezer. Increase the churning time to 50-60 minutes. You may add your favorite fresh, raw fruits such as sliced peaches or berries, or chopped nuts *after* ice cream freezer processing. Makes 4-6 servings.

---

[1] The FDA does not allow the use of the word "sweetener" for stevia, only "dietary supplement," which placates the artificial sweetener manufacturers. Stevia is available at the health food store.

Sugar-Free Ice Cream Float

Ingredients:

1 oz. non-sweetened cranberry juice (Knudsen's *Just* Cranberry works well)
5 oz. water
1/3 c. homemade sugar-free ice cream
Stevia powder to taste.

Creamy Cheese Cake
(Sugar-free)

This is another adaptation for a quick & easy carb-, sugar-, crust-, egg- free cheesecake many food allergy patients may enjoy. It isn't nutrient-dense, just a great way to satisfy "a sweet tooth." Husbands and teens who don't cook, will prepare it!

1 envelope unflavored, organic gelatin
1 c. water
2 pkgs. regular or Neufchatel, organic, low-fat cream cheese - organic[1]
1/4 tsp. stevia
1 tsp. vanilla
1/2 c. finely chopped nuts (optional), or
2 c. strawberries, blueberries or cherries - partially frozen (optional)

Sprinkle gelatin over 1/4 c. cold water in a small sauce pan; let stand 1 min. Stir over low heat until gelatin is dissolved. Blend with mixer in large bowl the cream cheese, stevia, and vanilla until smooth. Gradually add gelatin mixture and remaining 3/4 c. water and beat until smooth. Pour into flat bottom, glass dish for fast chilling. This dessert is delish with or without a topping. Cover with clear, plastic wrap. Chill approximately 30 minutes or more. Makes 4-6 servings.

---

[1] The Organic Valley Neufchatel (reduced-fat) cheese contains 30% less fat, or only 6 grams per 1 oz serving for those who prefer low fat. This cheese is cultured, not acidified.

Satisfying Buckwheat With Currants & Nuts

Served with a green salad or thick slices of red, ripe tomato and celery sticks, this is a great meat substitute occasionally The recipe is really easier than it may appear. Unlike beans, buckwheat cooks quickly and care should be taken not to overcook. Served it warm or cold.

Ingredients:

2 c. chicken or beef broth (homemade is best, cubes will do)
1 c. unroasted buckwheat groats
1/2 c. currants or chopped dried prunes
1/3 c. chopped nuts of your choice
1 T. thinly chopped green onions
1/4 - 1/2 tsp. sea salt
2 1/2 T. each oil & raw apple cider vinegar (see directions below)

Heat broth in a small pan (1 qt. or less) to boiling, stir in groats. Immediately reduce to lowest setting, cover with tight lid. Cook 12 minutes only. With large spatula, gently transfer to large pan or platter so as to cool quickly. Lightly turn with the spatula, then allow to cool for about 30 minutes. Add currants, nuts, green onions, and vinaigrette and gently toss. Makes about 3 cups.

Buckwheat has a small amount of complete protein. Drink a glass of milk with this meal to increase that amount.

Vinaigrette (or salad dressing)

Ingredients:

1 c. extra virgin olive oil
1/4 c. Bragg's raw apple cider vinegar
1–2 T. mustard of your choice (spicy brown mustard is good)

Place all ingredients in salad dressing container or small jar and shake well.

Chicken & Lentils

This meal-in-one simple dish, includes quality protein, complex carbs, healthy fats/oils, cooked tomato's lycopene; plus nutrient-rich okra's mucilage (demulcent that soothes and protects mucous membrane of lower intestine).

Ingredients

1 T. extra virgin olive oil (EVOO)
*2-4 lg. chicken thighs
1 c. chicken or beef broth
1 c. lentils
½ c. canned or frozen tomatoes
½ c. sliced okra (frozen is fine)
Salt

Place olive oil in 2 qt. pan. Add chicken, cover, and cook on low about 20 min. or almost done. Add broth, tomatoes, and lentils around chicken, leaving chicken on bottom and being sure lentils are in liquid, not on top of chicken. Cover and simmer about 15 min. (tilt lid if necessary to prevent boiling). Do not overcook lentils.

Remove chicken from pan, cool a minute, then remove meat from bone with paring knife, cut into bite-size pieces. Stir to combine ingredients. (Depending upon how much liquid you use, this may be enjoyed on the plate or in soup bowls.) Serves 3 or 4.

(One thigh = 25 g. protein, lentils provide additional protein, plus complex carbs.)

*Chicken breast may be used, however, the juice of thighs adds to flavor of this dish. If breast is used, add more broth.

Summer Low Carb Lunch Or Dinner Menu

This whole-foods meal provides an excellent variety of good fats for energy with the beef,[1] butter, avocado, and extra virgin olive oil. The broccoli phytochemicals may be protective of the lower intestine. The only carbs in this simple meal are in the avocado.

Broiled ground beef pattie (about 4 oz. ea.) Don't overcook.
Lightly steamed, buttered broccoli (LOTS OF IT!)
Salad of avocado, raw pumpkin (green) seeds, green onions, tomato, cuke.

Gently cube avocado halves and tomato into large pieces. Slice green onions, and peel and slice cuke. Add salad dressing.

Salad Dressing:

¼ c. extra virgin olive oil, 2 tsp. raw apple cider vinegar (or in proportions you prefer), tsp. of prepared mustard of choice, pinch of stevia (HFS), salt & pepper.

Avocado Macronutrients[2]

Calories	177.0 kcal
Protein	2.11 gm
Carbohydrates	6.91 gm
Saturated Fats	2.59 gm
Polyunsaturated Fats	2.04 gm
Monounsaturated Fats	11.21 gm

---

[1] Beef fat depends upon the amount added when the it is ground.
[2] Avocadotrees.com. Visit this website for lists of vitamins and minerals in this nutritious fruit.

Table of Acronyms Used

AA	Amino acid
ADR	Adverse Drug Reaction
AHA	American Heart Association
CAD	Coronary artery disease
CHD	Coronary heart disease
CVD	Cardiovascular disease
CLA	Conjugated linoleic acid
CRC	Colorectal cancer
EAA	Essential amino acids
EFA	Essential fatty acids
EPA	Ecosopenoic acid (Omega 3 EFA)
HFS	Health food store
MI	Myocardial infarction
PD	Prudent Diet
PUFA	Polyunsaturated fatty acid
SAD	Standard American diet
TFA	Trans fatty acids (trans fats)
WMD	Weapon of Mass Destruction

About The Author

For decades Sylvia W. Zook, MS, PhD, has taught and inspired many through her private practice, seminars, workshops, conferences, lecturing, eye-opening articles, newspaper columns, her own web site and countless other websites which publish her articles, international newsletter, e-zine and books.

With three family members having served as judges, as a child Dr. Zook developed an acute sense of justice. She was preparing to enter law school at the University of Alabama when lifelong health issues could no longer be ignored. She met the renowned W. M. Ringsdorf, DMD, research partner of Emanuel Cheraskin of the university's Birmingham medical research, who encouraged her to take an aggressive, proactive position, to begin her own research for her complicated case.

Later, when Dr. Zook sustained serious injuries in an auto accident, she redeemed that period of recuperation in alternative health care studies, then "hit the ground running!" beginning with John Jeffries, ND and the complicated dietary needs of *Candida albicans* patients (systemic fungal infections have emerged as a modern day, major health concern).

Ten years of higher education, 40 years of research, and Dr. Zook's years of practice have resulted in evidence-based bioavailable nutrition "tried in the fire." Before a lifelong brain tumor was finally diagnosed in 2004, the scriptural, scientific diet she writes about enabled her to maintain a fulltime practice, write and lecture extensively, with 60-hour weeks, for many years. Two physicians opined that diet and supplementation kept her alive and functioning unusually well all those years while working overtime to help others "falling through the cracks."

A growing body of evidence reveals that surgical patients' bodies heal much more quickly, and our bodies continually heal themselves, when two vital nutrients are provided in adequate amounts. In **Eatin' After Eden** – this knowledgeable professional reveals the critical nutrients, their unique bioavailable sources, and how much you need!

Education & Training:

Undergraduate studies – University of Alabama (Mobile, B'ham), School of Commerce & Business Administration; University of North Alabama, liberal arts and biology (total 6 years).

Postgraduate studies – Clayton College: MS & PhD in nutrition.[1]

Recognized as the leading college of natural health, Clayton College is #1 in the US in training natural health practitioners. Its aim is to produce skilled practitioners to serve clients with an educational empowering perspective. With a practical approach of teaching and consultation, individual clients are viewed as whole persons rather than sets of symptoms. Thus, this model embraces the belief that through imparting knowledge the practitioner empowers and motivates the client to assume greater personal responsibility for his or her health. After all, the Latin root of "doctor" – doctore' – means "to teach."

Continuing professional education:

In addition to 40 years of nutrition research, continuing professional education includes *New Perspectives In Nutritional Therapies; Improving Intercellular Communication in Managing Chronic Illness* with nutrition biochemist Jeffrey S. Bland, PhD, former Senior Research Scientist at the Linus Pauling Institute of Science and Medicine.

Dr. Zook also earned herbology certification from the former American Herbal Institute, applied enzyme nutrition with Howard F. Loomis, Jr., DC;[2] and participates in ongoing nutrition seminars with leading nutrition educators and clinical practitioners.

---

[1] The Amer Assn of Drugless Practitioners and the Amer Naturopathic Medical Accreditation Board accredit Clayton College. These are designed to meet the needs of unconventional education and are not affiliated with any govt agcy. The Ala State Dept. of Postsecondary Education licenses the college.

[2] FLACA, 21st Century Nutrition. Dr. Loomis studied under the noted authority and pioneer in enzyme research, Edward Howell, MD.

RESOURCES

Beyond Pritikin, Ann Louise Gittleman, MS, Bantam Books

Brain Power, Vernon H. Mark, MD, with J. P. Mark, MSc., Houghton Mifflin Co., Boston

The Cholesterol Controversy, Robert R. Pinckney, MD. "Read it from cover to cover," urges Mary G. Enig (*Know Your Fats*)

The Cholesterol Myths, Uffe Ravnskov, MD, PhD, New Trends Publishing, Inc., Washington, DC, 2000, www.ravnskov.nu/cholesterol.htm

Coconut Cures, Bruce Fife, ND, Piccadilly Books, Ltd., CO, Piccadillybooks.com

Coronary Heart Disease: the Dietary Sense and Nonsense, George V. Mann, ScD, MD (proceedings of the *Veritas Society*) Janus Press.

The Facts About Fats, John Finnegan, Elysian Arts, CA 90265

Fats That Heal, Fats That Kill, Udo Erasmus, Alive Books, BC, Canada, 1993

Goat Milk Magic, Bernard Jenson, PhD, Bernard Jenson Publisher, CA

Health Alert Newsletter, 5 Harris Court, N6, Monterey, CA 93940, 408/372-2103, www.healthalert.com, edited by Bruce West, DC. Excellent educational source for today's health challenges; use of whole-foods concentrations to support the body's healing work for various health challenges.

The Hidden Link Between Adrenaline & Stress, Archibald D. Hart, PhD, Word Pub., TX

Hypothyroidism: The Unsuspected Illness, Broda O. Barnes, MD, & L. Galton, Harper & Rowe; Broda Barnes Foundation, POB 98, Trumbrell, CN 06611

Integrative Medicine, A Clinician's Journal, POB 231655, Encinitas, CA 760/633-

It's All In Your Head, Hal A. Huggins, DDS, diseases caused by silver-mercury fillings

Know Your Fats, Mary Enig, PhD, Bethesda Press, MD

Life Without Bread, Christian B. Allan, PhD & Wolfgang Lutz, MD. Keats Pub. Excellent low carb treatise. Avoid processed foods in the carbohydrate table.

The Myths of Vegetarianism, Stephen Byrnes, PhD, see Weston A. Price Foundation's website.

Nourishing Traditions, Sally Fallon, MS, with Pat Connally & Mary Enig, PhD, ProMotion Pub, CA 800/231-1776

Nutrition and Physical Degeneration, Weston A. Price, DDS, Price-Pottenger Foundation, POB 2614, LaMesa, CA 91943-2614

Pasture Perfect, The Far-Reaching Benefits of Choosing Meat, Eggs, and Dairy Products from Grass-Fed Animals, Jo Robinson, Vashon Island Press, WA

Perfect Bones, Pamela Levin, RN, Celestial Arts, CA, excellent teaching on the use of whole foods concentrates for healthy bones. Price-Pottenger Nutrition Foundation, POB 2614, LaMesa, CA 91943-2614

www.price-pottenger.org. Whole foods nutrition from perspectives of Drs. Price & Pottenger.

Radiation Protection Manual, Lita Lee, Spillman Printing, CA, 1990

Salt: Your Way To Health, David Brownstein, MD, Medical Alternatives Press, MI, www.drbrownstein.com, 888-647-5616. This book provides important information on why it is so important to ensure adequate intake of unrefined salt in your diet.

SoyOnLineService.co.nz. This site provides an excellent educational service with information from many sources, including myriad scientific studies.

Springreen Products, Inc., N. Kansas City, MO. 816/221-3719 Source of unrefined cod liver oil, alfalfa-free green powder, whole foods vitamin C complex.

Standard Process 800/558-8740 For referral to a practitioner trained in the use of whole-foods concentrates.

The Whole Soy Story, Kaayla Daniel, www.wholesoystory.com/, the shocking truth about soy.

Zinc & Other Micro-Nutrients, Carl C. Pfeiffer, Keats Pub, CN

Order Form

I would like to order *Eatin' After Eden*....

Name:_____

Address:_____

_____

City:_____**Zip:**_____

Phone: (Home)_____**Work:**_____

Please send_____ copies @ $24.95 for a total of $_____

(Quantity discounts are available upon request.)

Pls. include $4.95 S&H for first book, $5.95 for
second book, and $6.95 for three or more. $_____

(Please calculate carefully, underpayment will be
returned, order unfilled.)

Allow 3 weeks for delivery.

Mail this order form with check or money order to:

Plumbline Publisher, P. O. Box 3743, Salem, OR 97302.

Note: Plumbline Publisher also accepts all major credit cards at:

http://www.EatinAfterEden.com/

Made in the USA
Las Vegas, NV
05 February 2022